MULTIPLE MEDICAL REALITIES

EASA Series
Published in Association with the European Association
of Social-Anthropologists (EASA)

MULTIPLE MEDICAL REALITIES

Patients and Healers in Biomedical, Alternative and Traditional Medicine

Edited by

Helle Johannessen
and Imre Lázár

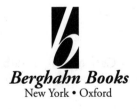

Berghahn Books
New York • Oxford

First published in 2006 by

Berghahn Books
www.berghahnbooks.com

© 2006 Helle Johannessen and Imre Lázár

Library of Congress Cataloging-in-Publication Data
Multiple medical realities : patients and healers in biomedical, alternative,
and traditional medicine / edited by Helle Johannessen and Imre Lázár.
    p. cm. -- (EASA series ; v. 4)
Includes bibliographical references and index.
ISBN 1-84545-026-4 (hbk.) -- ISBN 1-84545-104-X (pbk.)
    1. Alternative medicine--Cross-cultural studies. 2. Traditional
medicine--Cross-cultural studies 3. Medicine--Cross-cultural studies.
4. Healing--Cross-cultural studies. 5. Medical innovations--Social
aspects. 6. Medical technology--Social aspects. 7. Body, Human--Social
aspects. 8. Pluralism--Health aspects. 9. Medical anthropology.
10. Ethnology. I. Johannessen, Helle. II. Lázár, Imre. III. Series.

    R733.M855 2005
    615.8'8--dc22
                                                            2005040622

British Library Cataloguing in Publication Data
A catalogue record for this book is available from the British Library.

Printed in the United States on acid-free paper

Contents

List of Tables

List of Figures

Preface

Thomas Csordas

When good science makes an advance it pauses and turns to reacquaint itself with the modes of thought that immediately preceded it. Science orients itself with respect to these modes of thought, examines its connections, debts and disputes with them, decides whether it is operating at a different level of analysis and with respect to different interests, conceptualisations and subject matter. The present volume is a case in point of good science in this sense. It addresses medical pluralism, a founding concept of the field of medical anthropology. To the consideration of pluralism is added medical anthropology's more recent concern with body, self and experience. These articles demonstrate, with exceptional consistency, an assiduous attention to ramifying the interconnections between these two modes of reflection in medical anthropology, situating them as dialogical partners within the theoretical and empirical discourse of the field. In the process, both become refined and the field advances.

This observation can be elaborated as follows. Within any complex contemporary society, there exist a range of therapeutic alternatives ranging from biomedical treatment to religious healing, from highly technological therapies to casual folk remedies, and from professional treatment to informal treatment by family members. Such therapeutic alternatives are often based on very different cultural presuppositions, but in practice may be related to one another in the following four ways. First, they may be regarded as *contradictory* and incompatible, and hence in conflict or competition with respect to cultural legitimacy. Second, they may be regarded as *complementary* in the sense of addressing different aspects of the same health problem or category of problem, addressing a problem in a different but compatible idiom, or having an additive effect in alleviating a problem. Third, they may occupy *coordinating* positions within a total societal repertoire of health care resources, regarded as suitable for quite different kinds of problem. Fourth, they may be *coexistent* with contact or direct interaction, serving the differently defined needs of different segments of a population.

However, these relations do not necessarily define a structure. As practice theory has taught us, they may be understood as strategic options for defining the relative deployment of treatments throughout the course of any illness episode or healing trajectory. In other words, what a methodological standpoint grounded in bodily existence adds to an understanding of medical pluralism is experiential immediacy. In that immediacy the conceptual distinctions among medical systems and treatment modalities, distinctions that we may indeed find useful in mapping out situations of medical pluralism, can break down entirely. Here the descriptive language of pluralism is necessarily replaced by the existential language of self, intersubjectivity and the present moment. The intellectual polarity that is synthesised in these contributions thus reminds us that the core topic of medical anthropology is neither politics, economics nor political economy; neither biology, chemistry nor biochemistry, but the misery of those who are ill, the pity of those who become healers for those who are in misery, and the unwillingness by either to tolerate such pitiful misery.

Furthermore, as these studies conducted in all corners of the globe admirably show, pluralism may exist insofar as there are distinct practitioners who can be consulted for different kinds of healing, but also may exist within the practice of individual healers who possess expertise in a variety of therapeutic modalities of different cultural provenance – and both kinds of pluralism are to be distinguished from syncretism, in which different modalities or elements of therapy are combined in practice. Individual patients and healers may be highly eclectic in their choice of treatments or may be devotedly committed to one or more forms. The immediate experience of pluralism can be radically different for members of immigrant communities and those who are fluent with the cultural valuations placed on the alternatives available to them. Prior to all of this is the series of questions that has perhaps the most existential salience of all: what is the nature of the problem, how is it best defined, what are the criteria of diagnosis? Intuition and sensibility about these issues may determine initial choices among pluralistic options, or a disposition to consult one form of healing may predetermine how the inchoate distress of raw existence become shaped by the rhetoric of healing.

For Lázár and Johannessen, a principal motivation in having brought these contributions together is to argue that the proliferation of medical ideas, interpretations, nosologies and therapies across the globe is not evidence of a deep confusion in humanity's confrontation with affliction, a hit and miss effort to systematise an approach to affliction that 'gets it right once and for all'. The plethora of healing forms linked loosely by various degrees of elective affinity has a more radical implication in that it points to 'complexity in the body per se'. This articulates the truly intriguing promise of the synthesis between the study of medical pluralism and that of body, self and experience. The promise is that of elaborating the insight that the body is not only an organic entity, but the seat of a nuanced and multifaceted existence, a being-in-the-world.

In this sense the multiple realities of the volume's title are not fragments of reality that must be pieced together in order to construct a comprehensive understanding of illness and healing. Neither are they necessarily dimensions of reality that coexist in a manner analogous to the way string theory in physics posits multiple dimensions of the structure of the universe. For, in appealing to Alfred Schutz, they emphasise that 'It is the meaning of our experiences and not the ontological structure of the objects which constitutes reality'. In these essays, that in effect bring an always-relevant question in medical anthropology into a new age, medical pluralism clearly shows its transnational face, its postmodern modality and its experiential immediacy.

List of Contributors

Christine A. Barry, BA, Ph.D., Senior Research Fellow, School of Social Sciences and Law, Brunel University, United Kingdom

László Buda, MD, Ph.D., Associate Professor, Institute of Behavioral Sciences, Faculty of Medicine, University of Pécs, Hungary

Efrossyni Delmouzou, Ph.D., Lecturer P.D. (407180), School of History, Acheology and Cultural Resource Management, University of Peloponnese, Greece

Robert Frank, Dr, Research Fellow, Bielefeld Institute for Global Society Studies, University of Bielefeld, Germany

Anne Sigfrid Grønseth, Cand.Polit., Research Fellow, Department of Social Anthropology, Norwegian University of Science and Technology, Trondheim, Norway

Witold Jacorzynski, Ph.D., Professor, Centro de investigaciones y estudios superiores en antropología social, Sureste, Mexico

Helle Johannessen, mag.scient, Ph.D., Associate Professor, Institute of Public Health, University of Southern Denmark, Denmark

Michael Knipper, MD, lecturer, Institute of History of Medicine, Justus-Liebig-University, Giessen, Germany

Kristine Krause, MA, Ph.D. candidate, Junior Research Associate, Institute of Cultural and Social Anthropology, University of Oxford, United Kingdom

Kinga Lampek, Ph.D., Associate Professor, Institute of Applied Health Sciences, Faculty of Health Sciences, University of Pécs, Hungary

Imre Lázár MD, M.Sc., Ph.D., Institute of Behavioral Sciences, Department of Medical Anthropology, Semmelweis University, Hungary

Geoffrey Samuel, Ph.D., Professorial Fellow, Religious and Theological Studies, Cardiff University, United Kingdom

Gunnar Stollberg, Dr, Professor, Bielefeld Institute for Global Society Studies, University of Bielefeld, Germany

Tamás Tahin, MD, Ph.D., Professor, Institute of Applied Health Sciences, Faculty of Health Sciences, University of Pécs, Hungary

1

Introduction
Body and Self in Medical Pluralism

Helle Johannessen

Even at a glance, it is obvious that in all contemporary societies a variety of health care options exist and 'medical plurality' seems to be a common feature of today's world. The therapies available vary from one locality to another, and span from herbal medicines to biomedical treatments to psychological and spiritual forms of therapy. Different kinds of health care imply different techniques as well as different ideas of the body, health and healing. Research into these matters has been manifold, but two major theoretical trends stand out when considering approaches to the study of therapeutic options. One is based in the concept of medical pluralism; within this perspective pluralistic health care systems in Asia, Africa and recently also in Europe and the United States have been investigated, particularly with regard to the relevance of legal and socio-economic conditions for therapeutic practices as well as differences in explanatory models. Unrelated to the research in medical pluralism, there emerged in the 1990s in anthropology as well as in sociology and philosophy a growing interest in body and self, as well as the relation between body and self. This perspective emphasises the individual's creation of meaning in the midst of chaotic life events and acknowledges the importance of narratives linking health, body and sickness to the lifeworlds of everyday living, a theme that seems also to be important for an understanding of bodies and selves in medical pluralism.

The contributions to this volume as well as other research show that patients attend several kinds of therapy. Sometimes plural use of therapy is employed during a single sickness period in an eclectic way or according to certain hierarchies of resort, as demonstrated in Witold Jacorzynski's chapter on the case of a Mexican woman and in Kristine Krause's chapter on the case of a Ghanaian woman, both suffering from mental illness and employing biomedical treatment as well as spirit exorcism and prayer. At other times and/or places, sick persons seem to choose therapy according to what kind of problem they suffer, as Christine Barry reports from users of homeopathy in London, but it seems to be a general trend that sick people visit more than one kind of practitioner. The studies also show that practitioners of medicine apply a variety of therapies based in ideologies that may differ widely. In example traditional spirit therapy combined with western drugs, as demonstrated in Kristine Krause's chapter; or biomedical treatment and homoeopathy or Ayurvedic medicine, as shown in the chapters by Christine Barry, and by Robert Frank and Gunnar Stollberg. Patients and practitioners thus seem to relate to several ideologies of body, health and healing. This implies that one person may hold a plurality of explanatory models of the body, health and healing, with each being legitimised by a different worldview, and in view of the close relation of body and self, a discussion of plurality in selves and identities seems inevitable. At a workshop at 'The 7th Biennial Conference of EASA', we invited a discussion of these matters and urged contributors to combine insights from studies at the structural level of medical pluralism with insights from studies of individual people and their experiences of body and self. This volume contains contributions to the workshop, and this chapter suggests a theoretical frame for the discussion.

Any attempt to bridge the gap between phenomenological studies of body and self on the one hand, and studies on structural aspects of medical pluralism on the other, implies a conceptual framework that can encompass both levels. For this purpose, the distinction between the individual body, the social body and body politic as proposed by Margaret Lock and Nancy Scheper-Hughes in the 1980s (Scheper-Hughes and Lock 1987) is central. Bryan Turner's (1992) and Stephen Lyng's (1990) use of 'elective affinity' as a central concept for understanding connections between power, knowledge and the body complement this model. Elective affinity relates patterns in the multitude of body praxis with metaphors of body, self and sickness, as well as with policy and social institutions. New patterns emerge that connect but are at the same time dynamic and flexible.

Pluralism in medical structure

In the 1970s Charles Leslie's work on pluralism in Asian medical systems radically changed social science researchers' views of health care systems. Today it may be hard to understand how revolutionary Leslie's analysis was, but it really was a ground-breaking step. Leslie pointed to the coexistence of biomedicine and the traditional Chinese medicine system in China; and biomedicine, Ayurvedic medicine and Unani medicine in India; *and* to the fact that all of these traditions include major medical texts, educational institutions, and professionalised practitioners and treatment regimes (Leslie 1975, 1976). The Western idea of biomedicine (or Western medicine) as the only kind of sophisticated and well-developed medicine was shattered. Since Leslie pointed to the pluralistic character of health care in Asia, anthropologists have recognised the pluralistic character of health care all over the world. Research on medical systems and medical pluralism was alive and well established in studies of non-Western societies by the 1970s and 1980s. To mention just a few, one could point to John Janzen's study of medical pluralism in Lower Zaire (Janzen 1979); Emiko Ohnuki-Tierney's study of medical pluralism in Japan (Ohnuki-Tierney 1984); and Libbet Crandon's work on medical pluralism in South America (Crandon-Malamud 1991). A few studies of North American and European health care in the 1980s also turned to the concept of medical pluralism based on the notion of medical systems. Examples are the studies of Hans Baer, on the organisational development and social status of medical doctors compared to osteopaths and chiropractors in the United States and the United Kingdom (Baer 1984a, 1984b, 1987) and, more recently, Ursula Sharma's and Sarah Cant's research and discussion of complementary medicines in the United Kingdom (Sharma 1992, Cant and Sharma 1999).

The geographical move towards the West from the Rest illustrates that anthropological research from Third World countries has inspired new ways to conceptualise the home societies of Western anthropologists. In this case, concepts of medical pluralism and acknowledgement of the socio-cultural embeddedness of medicine that were developed abroad paved the way for acknowledgement and a scholarly discussion of various forms of medicine in the West. A recent renewed interest in medical pluralism repeats this geographical move. In 2002 a tribute to Charles Leslie and his impact on medical anthropological research in Asian societies was published (Nichter and Lock 2002), followed by an anthology on medical pluralism in the Andes (Koss-Chioino et al. 2003). The move is completed with the present volume, which has a substantial focus on European societies but which also opens up for a global scope, pointing to the universal character of the phenomenon.

Since Leslie's study of medicine in Asia, the notion of *medical systems* has been widely used in the research of medical pluralism but, as Irwin Press (1980) showed in a review of medical anthropological studies, the notion of medical systems has had very different meanings in different studies, and the notion of medical pluralism equally differs. Charles Leslie conceptualised only one medical system in each of the Asian countries he investigated, but each of these systems was pluralistic in the sense that a number of different medical traditions coexisted within it (Leslie 1975). John Janzen developed a different conceptualisation of medical systems in his study of medical pluralism in Lower Zaire, when he argued for the coexistence of multiple medical systems in the same community. According to Janzen, each system was made up of a body of practitioners sharing title, organisation and treatment modalities. With this perspective, Janzen was able to demonstrate the historical development of social organisations and legal rights for different kinds of practitioners in Zaire (Janzen 1979). A third way of conceptualising medical systems and medical pluralism is found in Emiko Ohnuki-Tierney's study of medical pluralism in Japan, in which she conceptualised three medical systems in coexistence: biomedicine, Kanpo medicine and religious healing. Each of these medical systems was comprised of a number of different kinds of practitioners who used different treatment methods but shared a common paradigm of health and healing (Ohnuki-Tierney 1984). The concept of medical systems and pluralism have thus been applied to health care in several studies since the 1970s, but some confusion and heterogeneity have prevailed as to what kinds of units to conceptualise as 'a system' and thus also with regard to the analytical level of 'pluralism'.

Before medical anthropology reached an agreement on the academic concepts of medical systems and systemic pluralism, however, the whole idea of systems and systems theory lost importance within the human sciences. As part of the postmodern sweep of the 1990s, the anthropological idea of medical pluralism became much more complex and unruly than indicated in studies from the 1970s and 1980s. Multiplicity and difference were acknowledged, but systemic order in the multitude was more or less rejected in favour of another theoretical trend that emphasised focus on the concepts of body and self.

Body and self in medicine

An important contribution to the conceptualisation of health, bodies and selves was provided by Margaret Lock and Nancy Scheper-Hughes in a paper from 1987 called 'The Mindful Body', which has since been republished in slightly revised versions several times (Scheper-Hughes and Lock 1987, Lock and Scheper-Hughes 1990, 1996). In this paper, Lock and Scheper-Hughes propose three conceptual levels of the body: the individual body, the social body and the body politic.

The social body has been the object of anthropological research at least since the 1970s. This conceptual level of the body refers to the symbolic representation in and of the body, i.e., idioms of the body shared by members of the same community (Lock and Scheper-Hughes 1996). Mary Douglas pioneered in this field by pointing out that in most cultures, the body is used as a social symbol. In Douglas' view, the body represents the nation state with hierarchies and different functional roles, openings and transgression of borders, or the body is likened with technologies of the society in which it lives (Douglas 1966, 1975). In the medical realm, a well-known example is the long hegemonic representation of the body as a machine separated from the self that emerged in medical clinics in the eighteenth century (Foucault 1975). More recently, a postmodern model of the flexible and specific body made up of cells attributed with 'social' characteristics well-known from Western societies has been revealed as dominant in Emily Martin's studies of immunology in the United States during the 1990s (Martin 1992, 1994).

The individual body refers to the individual's perception and conception of her body at a phenomenological level, where the lived body experience is in focus. This level was central in many studies of the 1990s. With the postmodern turn in the social sciences, focus turned to the individual, and in medical anthropology to individual bodies and selves, instead of systems and shared bodies of knowledge. The anthropological discourse changed: sick people were no longer considered as patients seeking help in health care systems, but became embodied selves holding embodied knowledge of their life and sickness experiences; practitioners were no longer representatives of different knowledge and treatment systems, but became detached experts holding disembodied knowledge of objectified bodies. A well-known example is the work on embodiment by Thomas Csordas, in which he proposes that whatever the body-self perceives is to be considered as true and embodied knowledge for the person in question (Csordas 1994a). By narrating talks with people attending spiritual healing sessions in a Catholic Church, he describes the body-self as it is experienced by these people, i.e., that pain has disappeared and a leg has been lengthened after being healed by a priest. To Csordas, this phenomenological experience of the body is as true as any scientific knowledge of bodily tissue or functioning (Csordas 1994b).

It is not that the scholars of the 1990s denounce medical systems, they simply do not consider the macro structures of health care. Their quest is a different one, aiming at documenting the knowledge of lay persons as real and existentially true ways of knowing. This enquiry may be seen as part of the postmodern war against science that swept through Western societies during the 1990s. It was a revolt against the hegemonic status of scientific knowledge, i.e., knowledge that was based on a detached, disembodied objectification of diseases, patients, nature and much more. In much postmodern medical anthropology, the plethora of experiences were acknowledged and discussed as part of existence and as part of the lifeworld of individuals, but not as part of larger social and cultural structures. Bodies and selves were likened to individual atoms fighting their way through life in a struggle for meaning, and cases of sickness were considered as quests for meaning. Anthropology by and large lost sight of the larger structures of power and shared knowledge, and thus also lost sight of the pluralism in systems of medical knowledge and treatment modalities, and the power struggles between them.

The Body politic refers to the social, political and economic regulations of bodies. Michel Foucault was a pioneer in connecting bodies and politics by pointing to the privilege of nation states to dispose of the bodies of citizens as they see fit in times of war and to choose what forms of aid to provide in cases of poverty and sickness (Foucault 1975). Foucault demonstrated the body-regulating power of regimes of knowledge, when considering legal rights and institutional priorities in medicine as well as in prisons and sexuality. Others have followed in his footsteps: Bryan Turner demonstrated the regulating powers of diets (Turner 1992), and Nikolas Rose convincingly argued that contemporary political regulation of the body works through the (illusionary) idea of the autonomous self with a free will and an ability to choose (Rose 1992). Many studies focusing on political aspects of bodies and selves have – like Foucault, Turner and Rose – explored sociocultural technologies of regulations (e.g., Martin et al. 1988). Others point to the economic interests connected with the regulation of the body (e.g., Baer 1989). An example of this perspective would be Michael Taussig's paper on 'Reification and the consciousness of the patient', which demonstrates how capitalist ideology has entered the patient-doctor relationship and inhibits a view of the patient as a person (Taussig 1992).

The three body levels are useful analytical tools, and Lock and Scheper-Hughes' paper as well as other studies have revealed a plethora of ways to experience, talk about and interact in relation to body and self, as well as a multitude of power relations that play on bodies and selves. Medical pluralism on a global scale with multiple symbolic representations of the body, a multitude of phenomenological experiences of health and sickness, and various modes of body regulation are thus amply demonstrated within this framework, but although pluralism at the three levels is recognised on a global scale, it is often neglected on a local scale. To my knowledge, the model has not yet been used as a theoretical frame for understanding patterns in the multiple and contradictory experiences and practices of body and self in which one individual engages, and which is found in any local society. It somehow seems to be anticipated that the population of a community shares a rather limited number of socially sanctioned body concepts and that the local body politic is concerned with promoting one main body construction. Emily Martin thus presents the idea of a national (or global?) transition from a cultural construction of the Fordist Body that reflects modernity and industrialisation, to a cultural construction of Flexible Bodies reflecting social values of postmodern late-capitalist society (Martin 1992).

The papers from this volume as well as data from my research among Danish patients and practitioners (Johannessen 1994) do, however, provide evidence of plurality on all three levels in contemporary small-scale societies. As do papers from the newer publications on Asian and Andean medicine (Nichter and Lock 2002, Koss-Chioino et al. 2003). We have evidence that individuals perform a number of bodily practices, and that a number of very different and yet locally acknowledged and shared concepts of body and self exist. On the political level of any one locality, one also finds a number of policies aimed at regulating bodies. Instead of a neat multilevel coherence of specific body politics represented in a local set of socially accepted and shared concepts of body and self, and experienced and practised in the lives of individuals, a messy reality with plurality at each of the three levels emerges.

Elective affinity in bodies and structure

This leads to the theoretical problem of how to conceptualise relations between the three levels or perspectives of the body. In the early version of their paper, Lock and Scheper-Hughes pointed to 'emotions' as the link between the three levels, but without specifying how emotions would link up the levels (Lock and Scheper-Hughes 1990). Later, they changed their argument and claimed that the three levels were linked through the 'body praxis' of each individual (Lock and Scheper-Hughes 1996), with bodily praxis expressing local social idioms of body and self, as well as local social organisation and politics of the body. In this optic, society and politics is embodied in suffering and distress in the sense that bodily praxis or distress may be the individual's only legal way of resisting unbearable social and political conditions. Somatisation, psychosomatics, premenstrual syndrome and mental illness may in this perspective be understood as socially significant indications of living condition (ibid.: 64–66). Although that explanation gives room for plurality, choices and different strategies among several possibilities of sickness and health care, it does not account for relations between specific forms of body praxis, specific body idioms and specific sociopolitical forms in a local pluralistic setting. Neither does it explain why certain forms of body praxis and certain body constructions are legally authorised and economically supported by national health authorities and others are not. How can these relations be conceived beyond recognition of the praxis of individuals, be they sick persons, doctors or politicians? Is it possible to reveal an implicit order connecting experiences, idioms and metaphors, and politics? Is it possible to discover a cultural stream or a pattern of patterns in the seemingly chaotic plethora? To answer such questions, we may turn to the works of the sociologists Bryan Turner and Stephen Lyng (Lyng 1990, Turner 1992) who independently of each other referred to the concept of *elective affinity* in explaining relations between praxis, knowledge and power.

Elective affinity originates as an analytical concept in the science of chemistry, where it refers to an inherent tendency of certain elements to combine with certain others and form new compounds. As Stephen Lyng has pointed to, the concept was later introduced to the social sciences by Max Weber to account for a relation between two social factors able to coexist in a stable relation because there is no opposition and tension between them (Lyng 1990: 138). According to Bryan Turner, most of Weber's discussion of rationalisation was informed by an argument of elective affinity in the relation between the logic of formal reasoning and specific interests of social groups (Turner 1992: 181). Weber was not concerned with the relation between body and knowledge, but Turner finds the concept of elective affinity important in the sociology of the body because it makes reference to the social and political context of knowledge and practices of the body (ibid.). Turner observes that certain politics have a tendency to be found with certain forms of knowledge and practice; this rule informs the conglomerates of politics, body knowledge and practice that exist in society. The three body levels, as proposed by Lock and Scheper-Hughes, may similarly be conceived of as connected by the principle of elective affinity. With regard to medical pluralism, then, the concept of elective affinity may explain connections between certain forms of praxis and knowledge and specific parts of local power structures. However, although Turner introduces the concept of elective affinity as 'the missing link' in connections across levels, he does not tell us exactly how and where to look for this affinity.

The American sociologist Stephen Lyng offers a more concrete conception of affinity in relations when he proposes that the concept of elective affinity refers to a dialectic relation in organising principles and thus to structure and patterns emerging in what he terms 'internal relations' (Lyng 1990: 52). Lyng demonstrates in his study of the biomedical health care system in the United States how the same organisational logic and principles permeate the knowledge dimension, the social dimension – both as microstructure (patient-practitioner relations) and as macrostructure (organisation of medical practice) – and relations to production (to the medico-technical industry). According to Stephen Lyng, the basic organising principle is to be found in the relation between consumers and providers of health, and he concludes that the essence of this relation is a fundamental opposition of interests between health consumers (patients) and health providers, with patients having an interest in holistic health care and providers an interest in reductionist health care (ibid.: 158). As a by-product of this analysis, Lyng also demonstrates the internal opposition of the organisational logic of many holistic therapies and the organisational logic of the social structure of biomedical health care institutions as well as the medico-technical industry. Lyng's study has some obvious and serious limitations, one of them being the rather simplistic picture he draws of biomedicine. Not all of biomedicine is governed by a reductionist principle, although one may consider the reductionist principle as dominant within biomedicine and in late-capitalist production, and as a dominant organising principle in various forms of praxis in Western culture.

In spite of limitations in studies of elective affinity in medicine, the concept of elective affinity provides a theoretical tool by which one can reveal an order in the local pluralism of the three body levels. Multiple organising principles are found on each level, and the relations between the levels can be conceptualised as being constituted by affinity or opposition between these organisational principles. The affinal relational patterns can, in a Batesonian framework, be conceptualised as patterns that connect; as patterns of patterns (Bateson 1988); each organising principle constitutes a certain structural pattern that is connected to the structural patterns of other entities or forms of practice through similarity or opposition.

Networks of body, self and power

The patterns that connect form new conglomerates and, inspired by Bruno Latour, these conglomerates can be conceptualised as actor-networks encompassing objects, knowledge, social institutions and persons (Latour 1993). With elective affinity in the internal relations between organising principles, different actors – in the broad sense of the word – link up and form collective bodies or networks. These networks are not closed, in the sense that each actor belongs to only this particular network. Rather, they emerge momentarily and more or less forcefully in the praxis of individuals. The theoretical concepts of patterns-that-connect and actor-networks provide for a conceptual order in medical pluralism without a return to a rigid conceptualisation of the coexistence of separate and independent sociocultural systems of medicine. Indeed, contributions to this volume as well as my own research on medical pluralism in Denmark make it clear that there are no such separate and independent medical systems definable by clear-cut boundaries between one system and the other. Rather, a number of networks on different levels and across levels can be found; networks that emerge in shared concepts and forms of praxis among laypeople and in clinical and educational institutions, but which stable and loyal populations of patients and healers never inhabit. On the contrary, persons, products, ideas and techniques transgress institutional borders all the time and yet, the movements and choices are not random. Rather, the existing medical pluralism can be conceptualised as open networks based on elective affinity in organising principles that come into existence through praxis, i.e., whenever someone acts, talks or writes on health or sickness. The starting point for any analysis of networks in medical pluralism is thus to observe what people do and say, and this gives the anthropological approach with participant-observation and interviews of all kinds a superior position for investigation in this field. The papers of this volume all contribute to this investigation, as all but one are based on fieldwork regarding the health care praxis of patients, families and healers of various kinds. All contributions focus on plural use of health care, and thus provide for a conceptualisation of networks in medical pluralism connecting the phenomenological lived body experience with shared and socially embedded knowledge and with body politics.

Body, self and sociality

While one finds representation of the individual, the social and the political level of body and self in all contributions to this volume, in Part I, the focus is primarily on the social implications of different conceptions of body and self. The papers, each in their own way, demonstrate the complexity and ambiguity of relations between sociality and representations of bodies; it becomes evident that there is no direct connection between specific idioms of the body, specific forms of treatment praxis and specific social identities.

Persons sharing social identity as biomedical doctors or homoeopaths, for example, may employ very different idioms of the individual body and forms of therapy in praxis, and specific forms of praxis may connect to networks formed by very different organising principles.

The first paper in Part I is atypical of the rest of the papers, as it does not involve participant-observation and in-depth interviews but is based on a regional representative survey on the use of alternative medicines in contemporary Hungary. It therefore does not provide for extensive elaboration of how patients and health care providers experience and conceive of body and self nor for elaborate discussion of networks emerging in Hungarian health care and yet, the numbers and correlations between parameters revealed in this study do suggest interesting issues and convey fundamental information on this matter. Apparently, a growing number of the Hungarian population turns to plural health care – in a pattern similar to that of many other European countries at this time. Among those who already have plural use, the body seems to be experienced as something problematic, since there is a strong correlation between chronic non-fatal disease and the use of alternative health care options as well as physicians of secondary care. This corresponds to data from other countries and has often been interpreted as a result of patients' pragmatic quest for relief. It may, however, be interpreted within the theoretical optic suggested above as an expression of elective affinity between unmanageable disorders of the body and plurality in health seeking. This may very well reflect an underlying elective affinity between the technical rationality dominating biomedicine and a rather limited number of bodily experiences. Those who experience bodily disorders that cannot be diagnosed and treated within the biomedical health care regime are doomed to try out alternative forms of health care on their own. For the time being, it seems that there are several networks in the health care of Hungary and that patients move between them to find forms of praxis and knowledge that match their bodily experiences. One network is dominated by the organising principles of a technical rationality and expert-based knowledge, and this network is supported by the state in a national health care system. Buda et al. suggest that physicians within the national health care system expand their repertoire of techniques and thus point to a more heterogeneous health care provided by the state and physicians as an adequate response to findings from their questionnaire survey on the use of alternative medicine.

The contribution of Imre Lázár disturbs the notion that the national health care system of Hungary is solely dominated by a technical rationality principle and connected to only one network. He demonstrates how the national communist authorities of Hungary favoured health care that complied with a technical rationality and yet, a number of traditional and more spiritually oriented healers have existed in Hungary during the many years of massive political support of technical biomedicine. Lately, forms of praxis from these traditions have been revitalised and included in the national health care system; and Lázár shows us an esoteric (hidden) side of health care, where psychologists in psychiatric wards engage in shamanistic drumming and journeys of the soul in their quest to heal those suffering from mental illnesses. He also shows us that well educated patients and families engage in ritualised forms of praxis with the aim to cure fatal physical diseases by work at a spiritual level. Lázár demonstrates very clearly that professionals, patients and families who are participating in the biomedical system also engage in forms of praxis that are not governed by a technical rationality, but rather by an existential rationality that emphasises spiritual relatedness and personal involvement. Some forms of praxis within the Hungarian nationally supported medical institutions thus form networks with idioms of the body as a spiritual being and healing traditions that have long been suppressed by national authorities; the heterogeneity proposed by Buda et al. seems already to be in emergence.

Kristine Krause demonstrates in her analysis of the treatment of a woman suffering from mental illness how Ghanaian medical doctors use pharmaceuticals in the morning and Christian rituals in the afternoon. This situation seems to be analogous to the Hungarian situation presented by Lázár, and one may conclude that it is just another example of the coexistence of a technical-rationality-network and an existential-rationality-network in the praxis of biomedical institutions. Krause goes one step further and demonstrates that even though pharmaceuticals and Christian healing may at first sight seem to represent different networks, they do at the same time show elective affinity with the same power elements, i.e., they both point to the hegemony of modernity and science. In the Ghanaian context, the apparent opposition between pharmaceuticals and spiritual healing is superseded by elective affinity between modernity, Christianity and pharmaceuticals, and, although pharmaceuticals link up with the medico-technical industry and spiritual healing does not, they nevertheless combine in a network whose governing organising principle is modernity.

From Germany, Robert Frank and Gunnar Stollberg present some very interesting observations that demonstrate elective affinity in forms of praxis and motives for their use among medical doctors. In an investigation of motives for the use of Ayurvedic medicine, homoeopathy and acupuncture among German medical doctors, Frank and Stollberg found that those who had pragmatic motives based in a wish to cure or ease chronic diseases mixed several forms of therapy in their practice, while those who held ideologies of holism or spiritualism in health tended to be purists using only one form of therapy, i.e., one of the alternative forms. This study clearly demonstrates the flexibility in network formation, as it is shown how specific treatment modalities, e.g., Ayurvedic medicine, is drawn into different networks depending on the context. In the mixers' use, Ayurvedic forms of therapy are linked with many other forms of therapy in a network governed by the quest to find solutions to chronic disorders, and the governing organising principle may thus be said to be pragmatism, i.e., it does not matter what idioms or sociopolitical structures are involved, as long as the treatment eases the patient's individual and phenomenological experience of the body. In the purists' use of Ayurvedic medicine, the links to Indian culture and philosophy are most important, and the praxis is thus part of a network that is governed by an organising principle of ethnicity. Christine Barry's study of homoeopathy in London similarly shows how one form of therapy is ambiguous in its relational embeddedness, as it is practised by laymen as well as medical doctors, within as well as outside the national health care system, and in a traditional way loyal to the principle of similarity as formulated by Hahnemann as well as in a more biomedicalised way. Barry distinguished between committed and pragmatic users of homoeopathy, and found that committed users actively sought out homoeopathy as a total treatment modality while pragmatics were often offered this form of treatment as one among several others by their general practitioner. The correspondence with Frank and Stollberg's findings in Germany is striking, with the difference being that in Barry's study, the network governed by pragmatism is seen from the patient's perspective, while the German study focuses on the practitioner's perspective. As in the German case, the alternative network for homoeopathic praxis among British patients is governed by organising principles of holism and spirituality.

Body, self and the experience of healing

The contributions to Part II take a close look at the processes individuals go through when exposed to different idioms and forms of praxis connected with their body. Sociality is also important in these papers, as all sickness episodes are articulated and to some extent developed as part of sociality. However, the focus is primarily on the phenomenological experience of body and self as changing when confronted with multiple medical realities and the implications this may have for the individual. Healing and relief for suffering are the aims of all efforts, but different forms of praxis imply different notions of healing and different relational processes.

Geoffrey Samuel offers a model of healing that is constituted in a relational network that encompasses 'mind, body, social and physical environment *as a whole*' and urges us to overcome traditional disciplinary vocabulary and analytical categories in order to understand the complex processes involved in healing. Samuel discusses childbirth praxis in a pluralistic North Indian setting and argues that while traditional birth rituals may (or may not) be proper from a purely biomedical view, they most likely make sense and inform birthing women and their families of what state the woman is in and how to behave in that state, and thus may ease the labour of the woman. A biomedicalised birthing in a hospital may be more appropriate in its own terms, i.e., in the provision of proper hygiene, but cultural and social distance to the birthing woman and her family may complicate the childbirth. Samuels thus provides a model that overcomes the dualism of body and mind in healing and provides equal space for the self in processes that in Western sciences are usually considered primarily physical and only secondarily cultural or mental. The individual body is, in this model, incorporated in the most literal (and corporal) sense in networks with praxis, idioms and politics.

Michael Knipper offers a case from Ecuador that likewise problematises biomedical ideas of how to instigate healing. He describes how he – a medical doctor – was called upon to provide treatment that from a biomedical point of view should not be effective and yet seemed to be of some help to the patient. He points to the meaning this intervention had within the local understanding of sickness, healing and persons in an explanation for the healing effect, and questions whether it is appropriate to talk about medical pluralism and differences in the phenomenological experience of the body when a biomedical form of praxis is incorporated in local understandings of the person. This case story makes us wonder what forms of networking the local use of seemingly universal forms of medical praxis may implicate. Does the patient in this case enter a global network organised around a technical rationality, or does the universal praxis of infusing sugar solutions enter a network organised around the local idea of 'samay' which is in no way restricted to the medical realm?

While Samuel and Knipper point to situations in which patients gain from a plural use of medicines, but within a conceptual framework that makes sense to the patients and their relatives, Anne Sigfrid Grønseth tells us about Tamil refugees in Northern Norway who experience a loss in their meeting with biomedical treatment. Being far removed from family networks and traditional Ayurvedic forms of treatment, the Tamils seek relief from social and physical suffering at the offices of biomedical doctors, but find that the doctors do not understand their pain and are not able to provide adequate treatment. The Tamils of this study are confronted with what might be called virtual medical pluralism, as the north Norwegian locality does not offer alternatives to the biomedical doctors, but in the memory of the Tamil refugees, Ayurvedic doctors, explanations and forms of praxis are alive and coexist with the biomedical reality they meet at the doctors' offices. This case demonstrates how diaspora is also at work in relation to health and healing, and how the individual experience of the body may connect to networks – including idioms, praxis and body politics – that may be found thousands of kilometres from the sick person.

Diaspora is also at work in the paper by Witold Jacorzynski's study of a Mexican woman suffering from mental illness, but in this case, the patient is actually moving between relatives living in different parts of Mexico in her search for a cure. This woman's experience is perhaps the most vivid example of a single person's exposure to multiple medical realities in this volume, as she consults a large number of practitioners including biomedical doctors, Christian healers, Indian curers, herbalists and many more. Her sickness is alternatively explained as a chemical disturbance, possession by the devil, possession by spirits, punishment for moral sins, etc., and the woman herself seems to be utterly confused as to what is wrong with her. There is no happy ending to this case, merely a demonstration of how people who all want to help the woman each contribute a little to more confusion about her case. Jacorzynski refers to William Blake's metaphor of a spider's web to illustrate the situation of the woman, a metaphor that links up very well with the network concept developed above. The various forms of praxis and idioms applied to this case connect to a number of networks organised around very different principles, including Godly punishment, spiritual relatedness, chemical balance and technical rationality, psychological suppression, and the fight between good and evil.

Whereas the woman from Jacorzynski's case is being pushed into different medical realities by family and friends, the young childless couple in a contribution by Efrossyni Delmouzou themselves struggle to present different medical realities to their families and friends in a constant attempt to keep up their social reputation. In this paper, Delmouzou demonstrates how rurally based Greeks are very selective as to how they explain current situations. In some social contexts, the lack of children in this particular family is explained as a deliberate choice informed by considerations of economy and career; while in other contexts, it is revealed that the couple does in fact try by all means to become pregnant. Whether the condition is expressed in medical terms or not seems to be dependent on the context and on what counts as morally sound, responsible and good behaviour in that particular context. The couple in this case does not seem to be confused in spite of the many different explanations they provide regarding the same conditions; this tells us that plurality in idioms and forms of praxis need not be a problem for the individual as long as control remains with the individual. The juggling around with multiple explanations – each pointing to different social positions and different forms of regulation of the body – connects the childlessness of the couple with many different networks, and, as long as the networks do not intermingle, the multi-networking seems to be successful.

Complex bodies and flexible selves

The contributions of this volume demonstrate that analytical order may emerge in the seemingly chaotic pluralism of perceptions and conceptions of body and self, in health care praxis and in political and institutional power, without regression to models of rigid and inflexible, closed systems. By considering pluralism at three levels of the body – the individual body, the social body and body politics – and as connected across these levels through elective affinity, medical pluralism is ordered into networks that are fluid and flexible. The individual patient or practitioner is not restricted to one network; persons as well as products and techniques move in and out of networks. An implication of this is that an individual's phenomenological experiences of body and self is flexible and may link up to different networks of praxis, knowledge and power as patients and practitioners move between the networks. The evidence of flexibility in experience and expressions of body and self among patients, families and those providing therapeutic interventions in localities from all over the globe calls for a concept of the complex body that incorporates the eyes that see the body and the discourse in which the body is articulated, as well as individual and political body praxis. The evidence from this research also provides for a concept of the flexible self in a constant struggle for social recognition, a struggle in which the complex body plays a significant role.

Networks are, however, not just analytical. They are very concrete in that the praxis of individuals at all levels have consequences for the individual body, the social body and body politics, as well as for personal, social and cultural life beyond health and sickness. Insight in complex bodies and flexible selves in open networks of praxis thus dismisses the innocence of medicine. It calls for an acknowledgement of the universal role of policies, clinical practice, institutions and research in shaping the individual's body-self into sociocultural sanctioned idioms of distress and healing.

The quest for relief and meaningful explanations seems to be universal, as does the interrelatedness of the individual body, the social body and the body politic. The plurality of discourses, institutions and forms of praxis available to the individual also seems to be a universal phenomenon. What differ from one locality to another are the particular discourses of distress and healing available, as well as individual strategies of manoeuvre among the pluralistic health options. In other words, patterns that connect the individual body-self, the social body and body politics and discourse can be found everywhere, but concrete configurations of the patterns and the individual hierarchies of resort are particular and locally situated. Moving between different networks, sick persons, families and health care providers juggle with issues such as personal identity and social, political and religious powers, as they seek solutions that may provide healing for the suffering body and at the same time provide for meaningful relations of the self.

References

Baer, H. 1984a. 'A Comparative View of a Heterodox Health System: Chiropractic in America and Britain', *Medical Anthropology* 8(3): 157–165.

——1984b. 'The Drive for Professionalization in British Osteopathy', *Social Science & Medicine* 19(7): 717–725.

——1987. 'The Divergent Evolution of Oesteopathy in America and Britain', *Research in the Sociology of Health Care* 5: 63–99.

——1989. 'The American Dominative Medical System as a Reflection of Social Relations in the larger Society', *Social Science & Medicine* 28(11): 1103–112.

Bateson, G. 1988. *Mind and Nature – a Necessary Unity*. Toronto, New York: Bantam Books.

Cant, S. and U. Sharma. 1999. *A New Medical Pluralism? Alternative Medicine, Doctors, Patients and the State.* London: Routledge.

Crandon-Mulamud, L. 1991. *From the Fat of Our Souls: Social Change, Political Process, and Medical Pluralism in Bolivia.* Berkeley: University of Los Angeles Press.

Csordas, T.J. (ed.) 1994a. *Embodiment and Experience: Existential Ground of Culture and Self.* Cambridge Studies in Medical Anthropology 2. Cambridge: Cambridge University Press.

———1994b. *The Sacred Self: a Cultural Phenomenology of Charismatic Healing.* Berkeley: University of California Press.

Douglas, M. 1966. *Purity and Danger: an Analysis of Concepts of Pollution and Taboo.* London: Routledge.

———1975. *Naturlige symboler [Natural Symbols].* Copenhagen: Nyt Nordisk Forlag.

Foucault, M. 1975. *The Birth of the Clinic.* New York: Vintage.

Janzen, J. 1979. 'Pluralistic Legitimation of Therapy Systems in Contemporary Zaire', in Z.A. Ademuwagun (ed.) *African Therapeutic Systems.* Honolulu: Crossroads Press, 208–216.

Johannessen, H. 1994. *Komplekse kroppe. Alternativ behandling i antropologisk perspektiv.* Copenhagen: Akademisk Forlag.

Koss-Chioino, J., T. Leatherman and C. Greenway (eds) 2003. *Medical Pluralism in the Andes.* London and New York: Routledge.

Latour, B. 1993. *We Have Never Been Modern.* New York: Harvester Wheatsheaf.

Leslie, C. 1975. 'Pluralism and Integration in the Indian and Chinese Medical Systems', in A. Kleinman (ed.) *Medicine in Chinese Cultures.* Washington D.C.: U.S. Government Printing Office, 401–417.

———1976. 'Introduction', in C. Leslie (ed.) *Asian Medical Systems. A Comparative Study,* Berkeley: University of California Press, 1–12.

Lock, M. and N. Scheper-Hughes. 1990. 'A Critical-interpretive Approach in Medical Anthropology: Rituals and Routines of Discipline and Dissent', in T.M. Johnson and C.F. Sargent (eds) *Medical Anthropology. Contemporary Theory and Method,* New York: Praeger, 47–72.

———1996. 'A Critical-interpretive Approach in Medical Anthropology: Rituals and Routines of Discipline and Dissent', in C.F. Sargent and T.M. Johnson (eds) *Medical Anthropology. Contemporary Theory and Method.* Westport and London: Praeger, 41–70.

Lyng, S. 1990. *Holistic Health and Biomedical Medicine – a Counter-system Analysis.* New York: State University of New York Press.

Martin, E. 1992. 'The End of the Body?', *American Ethnologist* 19(1): 121–140.

———1994. *Flexible Bodies: Tracking Immunity in American Culture from the Days of Polio to the Age of AIDS.* Boston: Beacon Press.

Martin, L.H., H. Gutman and P.H. Hutton (eds) 1988. *Technologies of the Self: A Seminar with Michel Foucault.* Amherst: The University of Massachusetts Press.

Nichter, M. and M. Lock (eds) 2002. *New Horizons in Medical Anthropology. Essays in Honour of Charles Leslie.* London and New York: Routledge.

Ohnuki-Tierney, E. 1984. *Illness and Culture in Contemporary Japan. An Anthropological View.* Cambridge: Cambridge University Press.

Press, I. 1980. 'Problems in the Definition and Classification of Medical Systems', *Social Science & Medicine* 14B: 45–57.

Rose, N. 1992. 'Governing the Enterprising Self', in P. Heelas and P. Morris (eds) *The Values of the Enterprise Culture. The Moral Debate*. London: Routledge, 141–164.

Scheper-Hughes, N. and M. Lock. 1987. 'The Mindful Body: a Prolegomenon to Future Work in Medical Anthropology', *Medical Anthropology Quarterly* 1(1): 7–41.

Sharma, U. 1992. *Complementary Medicine Today – Practitioners and Patients*. London and New York: Routledge.

Taussig, M. 1992. 'Reification and the Consciousness of the Patient', in M. Taussig *The Nervous System*. London and New York: Routledge, 83–109.

Turner, B. 1992. *Regulating Bodies — Essays in Medical Sociology*. London: Routledge.

Part I

Body, Self and Sociality

2

Demographic Background and Health Status of Users of Alternative Medicine
A Hungarian Example

László Buda, Kinga Lampek and Tamás Tahin

Societal processes are to some extent mirrored by transformation of the medical system of a given society. Among others, a symptom of the weakening of the predominant health care system with the underlying biomedical approach is exactly the appearance and spreading of different alternative forms of medicine spanning from traditional oriental medicine to distant energy healing, etc. In Hungary we are witnessing a significant increase of using alternative medicine (AM) both by visiting a practitioner and by buying, trying and applying herbal remedies and other alternative self-curing facilities. To understand the background and get a chance to discover reasons and patterns behind this phenomenon it is useful to obtain some empirical and quantitative data on the social reality related to it. Recently we have conducted a health-sociological research in Hungary, the aim of which was (1) to estimate the prevalence of, and likely, use of AM among the Hungarian population; (2) to identify demographic features of users of AM in order to refute the commonly held belief that AM in Hungary mainly serves as the last chance of desperate, credulous, naïve or poor people; (3) to investigate how AM use is associated with general health status; and (4) to obtain data about how AM is connected to the habits of turning to physicians and how we can describe as accurately as possible what actually is the role played by AM in the Hungarian health care system (Buda et al. 2002). Results from our study are provided in this chapter as particular examples of general trends in the distribution and use of alternative medicines in the contemporary West. Although the chapter is of a more epidemiological character than other contributions to this volume, we believe that the information is valuable because it outlines the quantitative distributions related to the use of AM, which is important background knowledge for the discussions carried out in the other chapters of this volume.

Use of alternative medicine (AM) in Europe and the United States

The popularity of AM (any sort of health/disease related intervention, method or system, that challenges the commonly accepted medical status quo or the bureaucratic priorities of the dominant professional health care in a given age and in a given society [Dossey and Swyers 1994]) has continuously increased for decades (Murray and Shepherd 1988, Sharma 1992, Fisher and Ward 1994, Eisenberg et al. 1998). The literature on the subject contains many publications that give an account of empirical investigations on several aspects of AM. A part of them examines making use of AM. Use may cover self-reliant utilisation of some alternative method, and/or calling upon an alternative healer (Eisenberg et al. 1993). The use of AM services may be studied according to different intervals (Sermeus 1987). The basic concern of some of the studies is the percentage of the population that has already turned to alternative providers during their lives (Donelly et al. 1985), others address use within a particular period (for example, ten years [Murray and Shepherd 1988], two years [Sutherland and Verhoef 1994], twelve months [Eisenberg et al. 1993, Northcott and Bachynsky 1993, Millar 1997], or two weeks [Blais et al. 1997] preceding the survey). Useful information is also yielded by measuring the number and frequency of use (Sharma 1992). Some publications discuss the utilisation of a wide range of AM procedures on samples representing the whole population (Fisher and Ward 1994, MacLennan et al. 1996, Eisenberg et al. 1998) or on a particular group of patients (for example cancer patients [Lerner and Kennedy 1992, Ernst and Cassileth 1999] or rheumatic patients [Ramos-Remus et al. 1999]). Other investigations concentrate on the use of one particular method or another, whether in general (e.g., chiropractice [Northcott and Bachynsky 1993]) or on a particular population (e.g., acupuncture in groups of people suffering from chronic pain [Riet et al. 1990]). In addition to users of AM there is a considerable proportion of those who, although they have never yet visited alternative practitioners, deem it possible in the future (Sharma 1992).

In Western Europe and the United States 20–50 per cent of the population uses alternative health services (Eisenberg et al. 1993, Fisher and Ward 1994). Data from Eastern Europe is much sparser, although the percentages of use may undoubtedly be estimated lower here (Fisher and Ward 1994). In Slovenia, for example, during 1997 the proportion of those who visited some alternative healer was found to be 6 per cent (Kersnik 2000). Sociological analysis of clients choosing some alternative treatment shows particular demographic differences as opposed to non-users. According to the surveys, people who visit alternative practitioners are mostly middle-aged and highly educated, with higher income (Sharma 1992, Fisher and Ward 1994). According to most publications, women are more inclined to turn to alternative practitioners (Bullock et al. 1997, Millar 1997), although some surveys found no significant difference between sexes in this respect (Eisenberg et al. 1993).

While the majority of publications discuss the presence of particular health problems in relation to the use of AM (Moore et al. 1985, Eisenberg et al. 1993) a minority examines the general health status of AM users (Blais et al. 1997, Millar 1997). The conclusions are mixed: according to some researchers AM users are generally less healthy and complain of more chronic health problems (Bullock et al. 1997, Millar 1997), notwithstanding that other studies, after having controlled demographic background variables, found no significant difference in health status (Blais et al. 1997). As regards visiting medical doctors, the data is again inconsistent. Some authors found that those who turn to alternative healers visit medical doctors more frequently as well (Sato et al. 1995), whereas others argue that AM users visit their general practitioners rarely as compared to the control group, rendering it probable that AM may play the role of an alternative to the primary health care (while no difference was found concerning secondary care) (Blais et al. 1997).

Alternative medicine in Hungary

Our earliest Hungarian data (Antal and Szántó 1992) come from a national representative survey from 1991, shortly after the collapse of the communist system. At that time 6.6 per cent of the adult population had used some kind of AM service and 39 per cent had shown some degree of openness toward future use. Those people having tried out AM were mostly middle-aged, urban and from the lower-middle class regarding their educational and occupational status. Those that were open to future use of AM were younger, urban, with higher education. A commonly held belief that AM users are hopeless people with terminal illness (especially with cancer), or people primitive and credulous enough to trust in these methods could be identified a decade before in Hungary (Antal and Szántó 1992). Since then, parallel with political and economic processes, the health care system and alternative care's role have changed. After a short period of uncontrolled pluralism, AM has been regulated by law and gained an accepted place as a collection of complementary methods besides official care. On the other side, the health status of people has also changed. People from the upper-middle class gained better health and found new possibilities of preserving their health condition while, those from the lower-middle class and under, were faced with worsening health status and poorer access to health care (Kopp et al. 2000). In such a context it seemed worthwhile to re-examine the present and future role of AM in Hungarian health care a decade after the political changes. Here we give a brief summary of our research together with some considerations and conclusions regarding the role of AM in relation to the contemporary dominant health care system.

The sample we observed was derived from the adult population of a county of Hungary (Baranya) by a multilevel, random selection method. The sample (N=2357) represented the population of Baranya county by age (between 28 and 69), type of settlement, education and occupational status. The data were collected by hired interviewers in 1999–2000.

As the definition of alternative medicine is controversial in circles of specialists (Pietroni 1992, Dossey and Swyers 1994) we may expect even less uniform interpretation by lay respondents of a sociological survey. In order to shed light on outlines of relations to AM as accurately as possible we investigated them along three dimensions. First, the dimension of use of AM offered by physician and/or non-physician was tested by two questions. The second dimension was the prospective inclination and openness towards turning to an alternative healer. These dimensions were statistically elaborated by logistic regression analysis. The third dimension consisted of two attitude statements concerning AM. By combining the three dimensions (six questions) an ordinal variable was constructed ('summarised relationship') ranging from 0 to 6, where 0 represented the most negative and 6 the most positive relations towards AM. This new variable has been analysed in a four step model by using the method of linear regression analysis. Independent variables comprised the demographic characteristics, the health status (measured by three parameters: (1) self-reported health status; (2) the total number of chronic diseases among which fatal and non-fatal ones were differentiated; and (3) restriction of activity due to health problems) and habits of visiting physicians.

Characteristics of the sample, along with the distribution of the dependent variables, are shown in Table 2.1. Out of all respondents 6 per cent have turned to physician alternative practitioners, and 10 per cent have visited non-physician alternative practitioners. The total value of 'use' proved to be 13 per cent. Prospectively 30 per cent would turn to physician alternative practitioners, and 21 per cent would turn to non-physician alternative practitioners. The total value of 'openness' proved to be 32 per cent. 55 per cent did not agree with the statement that most alternative healers' job is only moneymaking while 41 per cent admitted that such methods may help even in cases deemed incurable.

The factors influencing the *use* of alternative care according to logistical regression analysis are: lower age, higher education, the prevalence of more chronic but not fatal illnesses, more frequent visiting of physicians and less frequent visits to general practitioners (Table 2.2). The likelihood of having already turned to some alternative healer is 1.7 times higher for the youngest group than for the oldest group, and 2.2 times higher for white collar workers compared to those with lower education. The connection between the number of chronic (non-fatal) illnesses on the one hand and 'use' on the other is highly significant: those who have four or more such illnesses were five times more likely to visit some alternative healer than those who had none at all. The connection between the frequency of visiting physicians and AM use is similarly close: those who visited some physician more than six times in the preceding twelve months are 3.5 times likelier to have also used some kind of alternative care than are those who had not seen a doctor at all in this period. Concerning visits to general practitioners, this connection reverses: those who visit their GP more frequently are less likely to use alternative providers' services.

With regards to prospective *openness* to use AM, the impacts of age, occupational status, type of settlement, self-reported health status, the number of chronic, non-fatal illnesses and number of times visiting a physician proved to be statistically significant (Table 2.2). For 'openness' the role of lower age proved to be even more powerful than in the case of 'use'. Higher educational status is also a factor that increases likelihood, white collar workers being 1.6 times more inclined to use AM in the future than unskilled blue collar workers. By examining the position in the hierarchy of settlements, it is striking that the values of 'openness' are primarily high among the inhabitants of the regional centre (Pécs): here the ratio of likelihood is 2.4 times that of the smallest settlements. The better someone judges his/her own health status the easier it is for him/her to imagine turning to an alternative healer in the future: those who deem themselves having good or excellent medical condition are 1.7 times more inclined to be open than those who judge their health conditions poor. A rise in the number of chronic, non-fatal diseases is associated with a more distinct openness, but not as closely as in the case of use. In the regression analysis of 'openness' the measures of visiting medical doctors show a pattern similar to the case of 'use': a higher number of visits to any kind of physician and lower number of visits to general practitioners is significantly connected to a higher degree of 'openness'.

The linear regression analysis – concerning the aggregate index of the relations to AM ('use' *plus* 'openness' *plus* 'attitudes') according to the examined independent variables – was executed in four steps (Table 2.3). Among the basic demographic variables initially introduced into the regression model (sex, age, education), lower age and higher education are connected with a positive relation; however, sex makes virtually no difference. Introducing additional important demographic characteristics into the model, in the next step higher educational status, higher income and the type of settlement (to the advantage of towns) have a significant effect, while the significance of education fades (it is replaced by the influence of the former factors). By introducing health status into the model, 'better' self-reports and a greater number of chronic diseases (confined only to non-fatal ones) can be identified. The linear regression analysis corroborates that the relation to AM, having controlled by the demographic and health status parameters, correlates positively with the frequency of visiting doctors and negatively with visiting general practitioners. Among all cases of visiting doctors, those with the purpose of healing were indifferent while those with the purpose of prevention and control showed a positive relation to the dependent variable.

Integrative future prospects

Now it is time to consider whether our results can add something to the debate concerning AM or can strengthen the findings of international research in other Western countries during the last decades. While AM is considered to be expanding worldwide, the process has special dynamics in communist countries where it was illegal until one and a half decades ago. According to our results AM probably continues to spread in Hungary as judged by a comparison of national data from 1991 (Antal and Szántó 1992) with our regional data from 1999–2000. However, in Hungary, as compared to most of the Western European countries, the use and the openness rates are still lower (Fisher and Ward 1994). The recent history and the present economic and cultural status of the country can offer evident explanations to this phenomenon. Even though the legal regulation of the field came into existence in 1997 when AM was considered a legal 'health care activity' with the name of 'complementary medicine', people do still not have much information on the subject or about the actual possibilities of turning to AM healers. Thanks to the advertisements and available readings herbal products and other self-used 'alternative' therapies seem to become more and more popular in Hungary.

A greater proportion of our sample has already turned to *non-physician alternative healers*, whereas more participants leave open the possibility of a prospective use of alternative services by a *medical doctor*. This may be a signal for a possibility regarding the extension of use of AM in Hungary to be expected in the latter direction. In the past decade, some strange and scientifically questionable methods (e.g., healing with 'energies' from different sources) have gained extreme popularity for a while. Also the massmedia has assisted this process. Nowadays, people are less enthusiastic and more careful. AM users try out new directions but still trust (or try to trust) doctors. On the other side, medical doctors should learn a lot more about AM and the societal processes behind it. To accept their patients' ambitions to try out other methods or to visit other healers should be accepted and tolerated or rejected in a very careful and professional manner. Knowing how vulnerable the doctor-patient relationship is nowadays it seems to be extremely advisable for family doctors to learn more about AM in general and about the AM providers in the neighbourhood.

In relating to AM we found no significant sexdifferences in our study – a result that deviates from most of the data in the international literature. The reasons for these interesting findings are to be investigated in further research. The role of lower age is shown in both 'use' and 'openness'. It is primarily salient in the case of 'use' since younger people, despite the lower number of years of their lives, have turned to some alternative healer more often than older ones. This kind of connection between lower age and AM sympathy is well known in the international literature and refers to the general readiness of young people to 'enter the unknown' or rather, older people's inclination to keep a distance from uncertainty.

As in Western Europe, AM in Hungary attracts people of higher social status. Given this finding, the belief that AM has the greatest effect on 'primitive' and credulous people is not borne out in reality. In this respect, use of AM in Hungary reflects that of other Western European countries, so we are now witnessing a sort of 'closing of ranks' with the West. At the same time, the fact that the upper quarter of the income status groups significantly deviates in a positive direction, while the lower three quarters are virtually uniform in this respect, may be a specific Hungarian characteristic. Summing up, those having a higher position in social hierarchy have better health status on one side and have easier access to AM on the other, which may again, serve their health promotion. This in other words means that the gap, continuously increasing between the higher and the lower classes of Hungarian society with respect to their health status, is, among others, nourished by AM.

The conceptual distinction between visiting alternative practitioners on the one hand and openness to it on the other seems to be reasonable, as higher education in the first case and higher occupational status plus a higher position in the hierarchy of settlements in the second case were found to be significant background factors. The latter has an important role in the formation of the 'summarised relationship' also, indicating that AM would spread more intensively in more populated communities of Hungary. It seems to be true all around the world despite the fact that AM has its traditional roots in provincial rather than in urban milieu.

The connection between AM and health status was examined in several dimensions. The self-reported health status is not associated with the use of AM whereas it is positively connected to 'openness' and 'summarised relationship'. This may be a signal of the fact that the need for preserving health – as documented in the international literature (Furnham and Smith 1988, Furnham and Kirkcaldy 1996) – may play a role in maintaining the possibility of prospective use and in the formation of a positive attitude. Interviews with clients visiting AM practitioners also back up this statement since many of them clearly identified health prevention when listing their goals of the given visit. If the significance of AM in health prevention and promotion could be empirically proven, perhaps health politics could also react to that in a more conscious and generous way, e.g., supporting AM instead of restricting the field or incorporating some and rejecting other forms of AM on so called 'scientific grounds'.

According to our data – and in accordance with the literature (Bullock et al. 1997, Millar 1997) – we may suggest that a preference of alternative healing is unambiguously connected to the presence of more non-fatal illnesses but it is independent of fatal harms and states of restricted activity. The reason of this fact may be that AM offers an alternative to those people who suffer from long-lasting, unpleasant but not threatening illnesses, for it is a situation in which one is hardly exposed to risk by the use of AM, but may get a new chance of a possible improvement. In cases of more serious, life-threatening health problems, patients are inclined to lean on special medical care and would not take the risk of using some alternative treatment. This may remain true in spite of the fact that there are some fatal diseases (mainly illnesses difficult to cure or deemed to be incurable like cancer or AIDS) that lead people to visit alternative providers in greater proportions (Lerner and Kennedy 1992, Bullock et al. 1997, Ernst and Cassileth 1999), but their statistical weight remains minimal as opposed to the non-fatal, chronic states. In such cases the risk of seeking alternatives diminishes again as a consequence of despair and hopelessness. Our results give a statistical confirmation of Nagata's model on the adequacy of the different medical approaches, parallel with the severity phase of the illness, saying that the biomedical approach is effective mainly in the acute, organically obvious phase of an illness, while traditional oriental medicine and psychosomatic approaches are much more adequate in the first, preorganic, and the third, chronic or terminating phases (Nagata 1995).

Consistent with the result of surveys already known (Sato et al. 1995, Blais et al. 1997), it was found that alternative healing is more preferred by those who visit medical doctors more frequently too. This finding supports the idea that people do not necessarily think in terms of mutually exclusive alternatives (as is implied by the term 'alternative medicine'). On the other hand, our data supports the notion that in the field of primary care AM can work as a kind of alternative (Blais et al. 1997), as the frequency of visits to general practitioners showed a negative connection with all our three dependent variables. Apart from the fact that the higher rate of visiting physicians is due to the use of secondary care, it may bear importance that those who visit medical doctors with the purpose of prevention and control are more attracted by AM than those visiting medical doctors for the purpose of healing. This latter result may also indicate that people who would prefer AM tend to use available possibilities of preventing illnesses and maintaining good health more actively while they entrust their healing to traditional medical care to a lower extent. Along with other factors, skepticism towards official health care (Furnham and Smith 1988, Furnham and Forey 1994, Furnham and Kirkcaldy 1996) may contribute to this, as well as the abundantly documented unfavourable changes in the doctor-patient relationship (Hewer 1983).

It is recognised in the developed countries that a kind of good working integration between academic medicine and alternative medicine is urgently needed. However, the form of it is still unclear and differs from country to country. In Hungary, with the legal regulation, the overwhelming part of AM has gone underground. With the help of the law, official medicine incorporated a small, and marginalised a large part of AM. Out of the estimated fifteen thousand practitioners less than a thousand alternative practitioners requested a license five years after. Obviously, this kind of regulation can only partly serve the interest of the help seekers. The question is clear, the answer is 'under construction'.

Acknowledgements

The research was funded by OTKA (F023689, F029839).

References

Antal, Z.L. and Z. Szántó. 1992. 'A természetgyógyászat és az orvostudomány konfliktusa' [Conflicts between Scientific and Alternative Medicine], in *Leltár (MTA kiadvány)*, 79–92.

Blais, R., A. Maiga and A. Aboubacar. 1997. 'How Different are Users and Non-users of Alternative Medicine?', *Canadian Journal of Public Health* 88(3): 159–162.

Buda, L., K. Lampek and T. Tahin. 2002. 'The Role of Alternative Medicine in Health Status and Health Care System in Hungary', *Orv Hetil* 142(17): 891–896.

Bullock, M.L., A.M. Pheley, T.J. Kiresuk, S.K. Lenz and P.D. Culliton. 1997. 'Characteristics and Complaints of Patients Seeking Therapy at a Hospital-based Alternative Medicine Clinic', *Journal of Alternative and Complementary Medicine* 3(1): 31–37.

Donelly, W.J., J.E. Spykerboer and Y.H. Thong. 1985. 'Are Patients Who Use Alternative Medicine Dissatisfied With Orthodox Medicine?', *Medical Journal of Austria* 142(10): 539–541.

Dossey, L. and J.P. Swyers. 1994. 'Introduction', in B.M Berman and D.B. Larson, (eds) *Alternative Medicine: Expanding Medical Horizons*. Virginia: Chantilly. xxxvii–xlviii.

Eisenberg, D.M., R.B. Davis, S.L. Ettner, S. Appel, S. Wilkey and M.V. Rompay. 1998. 'Trends in Alternative Medicine Use in the United States, 1990–1997', *Journal of American Medical Association* 280(18): 1569–1575.

Eisenberg, D.M., R.C. Kessler, C. Foster, F.E. Norlock, D.R. Calkins and T.L. Delbanco. 1993. 'Unconventional Medicine in the United States', *New England Journal of Medicine* 28: 246–252.

Ernst, E. and B.R. Cassileth. 1999. 'The Prevalence of Complementary/alternative Medicine in Cancer: a Systematic Review', *Cancer* 83(4): 777–782.

Fischer, P. and A. Ward. 1994. 'Complementary Medicine in Europe', *British Medical Journal* 309: 107–111.

Furnham, A. and J. Forey. 1994. 'The Attitudes, Behaviors and Beliefs of Patients of Conventional vs. Complementary (Alternative) Medicine', *Journal of Clinical Psychology* 50(3): 458–469.

Furnham, A. and B. Kirkcaldy. 1996. 'The Health Beliefs and Behaviours of Orthodox and Complementary Medicine Clients', *British Journal of Clinical Psychology* 35(1): 49–61.

Furnham, A. and C. Smith. 1988. 'Choosing Alternative Medicine: a Comparison of the Beliefs of Patients Visiting a General Practitioner and a Homeopath', *Social Science & Medicine* 26(7): 685–689.

Hewer, W. 1983. 'The Relationship between the Alternative Practitioner and His Patient', *Psychotherapy and Psychosomatics* 40(1–4): 172–180.

Kersnik, J. 2000. 'Predictive Characteristics of Users of Alternative Medicine', *Schweizerische Medizinishe Wochenschrift* 130(11): 390–394.

Kopp, M.S., Á. Skrabski and S. Szedmák. 2000. 'Psychosocial Risk Factors, Inequality and Self-rated Morbidity in a Changing Society', *Social Science & Medicine* 51: 1350–1361.

Lerner, I.J. and B.J. Kennedy. 1992. 'The Prevalence of Questionable Methods of Cancer Treatment in the United States', *Canadian Cancer Journal of the Clinic* 42(3): 181–192.

MacLennan, A.H., D.H Wilson and A.W. Taylor. 1996. 'Prevalence and Costs of Alternative Medicine in Australia', *The Lancet* 347(9001): 569–573.

Millar, W.J. 1997. 'Use of Alternative Health Care Practitioners by Canadians'. *Canadian Journal of Public Health* 88(3): 154–158.

Moore, J., K. Phipps and D. Marcer. 1985. 'Why do People Seek Treatment by Alternative Medicine?', *British Medical Journal* 290: 28–29.

Murray, J. and S. Shepherd. 1988. 'Alternative or Additional Medicine? A New Dilemma for the Doctor', *Journal of the Royal College of General Practitioners* 38: 511–514.

Nagata, K. 1995. 'Comprehensive Medicine Based on Whole Person Medicine – Its Philosophy, Methodology and Strategy', *Dialogue and Universalism* 2: 45–52.

Northcott, H.C. and J.A. Bachynsky. 1993. 'Current Utilization of Chiropractic: Prescription Medicines, Nonprescription Medicines and Alternative Health Care', *Social Science & Medicine* 37(3): 431–435.

Pietroni, P. 1992. 'Beyond the Boundaries: Relationship between General Practice and Complementary Medicine', *British Medical Journal* 305: 564–566.

Ramos-Remus, C., S. Gutierrez-Urena and P. Davis. 1999. 'Epidemiology of Complementary and Alternative Practices in Rheumatology', *Rheumatic Disease Clinics of North America* 25(4): 789–804.

Riet, G., J. Kleijnen and P. Knipschild. 1990. 'Acupuncture and Chronic Pain: a Criteria-based Meta-analysis', *Journal of Clinical Epidemiology* 43(11): 1191–1199.

Sato, T., M. Takeichi, M. Shirahama, T. Fukui and J.K. Gude. 1995. 'Doctor-shopping Patients and Users of Alternative Medicine among Japanese Primary Care Patients', *General Hospital Psychiatry* 17: 115–125.

Sermeus, G. 1987. *Alternative Medicine in Europe. A Quantitative Comparison of the Use and Knowledge of Alternative Medicine and Patient Profiles in Nine European Countries.* Brussels: Belgian Consumer's Association.

Sharma, U. 1992. *Complementary Medicine Today – Practitioners and Patients.* London and New York: Routledge.

Sutherland, L.R. and M.J. Verhoef. 1994. 'Why Do Patients Seek a Second Opinion or Alternative Medicine?', *Journal of Clinical Gastroenterology* 19(3): 194–197.

Table 2.1 *Main demographic variables and rates of 'use' and 'openness'*

	distribution		'use'	'openness'
	N	%	%	%
Sex				
Male	1082	45.9	11.7	29.8
Female	1275	54.1	14.2	33.1
Age				*
28–39 years	614	26.1	14.0	38.1
40–49 years	673	28.6	13.7	34.6
50–59 years	580	24.6	12.8	30.7
60–69 years	490	20.8	11.0	20.2
Education			*	*
Primary school	804	34.1	9.6	21.0
Trade school	666	28.3	10.3	30.5
High school	532	22.6	17.9	37.9
College or university	355	15.1	18.5	46.0
Marital status				
Never married	311	13.2	10.6	30.9
Married	1784	75.4	13.4	32.6
Divorced, widow, separated	262	11.1	13.4	25.2
Occupational status			*	*
White collar worker with degree	271	11.5	17.2	44.3
White collar worker without degree	502	21.3	17.2	40.2
Skilled manual worker	812	34.5	12.0	31.3
Unskilled manual worker	772	32.8	10.0	21.8
Income status				*
Above average	547	23.2	15.1	37.8
Average or below average	1810	76.8	12.4	29.7
Type of settlement			*	*
Above 100,000 inhabitants	1098	46.6	15.4	40.7
10–100,000 inhabitants	436	18.5	13.4	25.7
2–10,000 inhabitants	482	20.4	11.0	25.7
Below 2000 inhabitants	341	14.5	7.6	17.9
Total	2357	100	13.0	31.6

= Sig.<0.001

Table 2.2 *Logistic regression analysis of 'use' and 'openness' (N = 2357)*

Variables	'use'		'openness'	
	OR	Sig	OR	Sig
Sex				
Male	1		1	
Female	0,98		1,06	
Age		*		*
60–69 years	1		1	
50–59 years	1,02		1,53	
40–49 years	1,29		1,79	
28–39 years	1,71	**	2,23	**
Education		**		
Primary school	1		1	
Trade school	1,06		1,02	
High school	1,86	*	1,06	
College or university	2,20	*	1,39	
Occupational status				*
Unskilled manual worker	1		1	
Skilled manual worker	1,06		1,28	
White collar worker without degree	1,12		1,59	**
White collar worker with degree	1,05		1,39	
Type of settlement				***
Below 2000 inhabitants	1		1	
2–10,000 inhabitants	1,46		1,52	*
10–100,000 inhabitants	1,41		1,27	
Above 100,000 inhabitants	1,54		2,36	***
Self reported health status				**
Poor	1		1	
Fair	0,92		1,19	
Good	0,81		1,72	**
Excellent	1,47		1,77	*
Chronic, non-fatal illnesses		***		**
None	1		1	
1 illness	2,04	***	1,33	*
2–3 illnesses	3,07	***	1,63	***
More illnesses	4,89	***	1,59	**

Table 2.2 *continued*

Variables	'use'		'openness'	
	OR	Sig	OR	Sig
Number of visits to physicians in the preceding 12 months (total)		***		***
No visits	1		1	
1–2 visits	2,11	**	1,78	**
3–6 visits	2,74	**	2,42	***
7 or more visits	3,55	***	2,93	***
Number of visits to GP's in the preceding 12 months		**		**
No visits	1		1	
1–2 visits	0,71		0,78	
3–6 visits	0,42	***	0,52	***
7 or more visits	0,48	**	0,49	***
	Goodness of fit: Model Chi-square =145,2 df=25 Sig.<0.001		*Goodness of fit: Model Chi-square =223,3 df=25 Sig.<0.001*	

*= Sig.<0.05 **= Sig.<0.01 ***= Sig.<0.001

Table 2.3 *Linear regression analysis of 'summarised relationship' (N = 2357)*

Model		B	Beta	Sig	R²
1	Constant	3,196		,000	,035
	Sex	,103	,035	,102	
	Age.	,019	,143	,000	
	Education	,050	,099	,000	
2	Constant	2,550		,000	,070
	Sex	,073	,025	,240	
	Age	,020	,151	,000	
	Education	−,008	−,016	,520	
	Marital status	,089	,026	,217	
	Occupational status	,170	,115	,000	
	Income	,188	,054	,013	
	Hierarchy of settelement	,169	,129	,000	
3	Constant	2,495		,000	,079
	Sex	,033	,011	,599	
	Age	,022	,162	,000	
	Education	−,008	−,016	,511	
	Marital status	,095	,028	,183	
	Occupational status	,160	,108	,000	
	Income	,180	,051	,018	
	Hierarchy of settlement	,166	,127	,000	
	Self-reported health status	,110	,057	,026	
	Number of fatal chronic illnesses	−,008	−,003	,905	
	Number of non-fatal chronic illnesses	−,379	−,125	,000	
	Activity-restriction	−,045	−,014	,507	
4	Constant	2,691		,000	,088
	Sex	−,009	−,003	,885	
	Age	,021	,156	,000	
	Education	−,009	−,019	,449	
	Marital status	,095	,027	,184	
	Occupational status	,153	,103	,000	
	Income	,186	,053	,014	
	Hierarchy of settlement	,152	,117	,000	
	Self-reported health status	,137	,072	,007	
	Number of fatal chronic illnesses	,052	,018	,471	
	Number of non-fatal chronic illnesses	−,335	−,110	,000	
	Activity-restriction	−,039	−,012	,561	
	Frequency of visiting physician (total)	−,146	−,110	,024	
	Frequency of visiting GP	,165	,129	,001	
	Frequency of visiting physician (curative)	−,115	,060	,107	
	Frequency of visiting physician (preventive)	−,111	−,061	,032	

3

Táltos Healers, Neoshamans and Multiple Medical Realities in Postsocialist Hungary

Imre Lázár

The conflict between Western biomedicine as the politically dominant health system based on bioreductionist assumptions and unconventional medicine with its wide eclectic syncretism reflects the cultural tension of the modern and postmodern. Hungary is itself undergoing a rite of passage from socialist modernism to globalised postmodernity. This liminality describes a situation of incomplete transition, a transformation in which elements of the old and the new coexist side by side without much integration (Schopflin 2002). This cultural transition has made people pay the high price of ill health, as self-destructive cycles arose in the midst of cultural and socioeconomic transition, depressive symptomatology and health in a rapidly polarising society (Kopp 2000). As rituals always accompany transitions from one social world to another, in this 'postmodern turn' we may rediscover the rituals and their culturally transformative role in unconventional medicine, where – citing Turner (1982: 86) – 'dismembering may be a prelude to re-membering'. It is more pronounced in those who express their frustrations and helplessness in somatisation or illness. Illness itself is a heightened state of receptivity in which a patient calls for another style of knowing in the context of the ultimate values of that patient's community. The human body offers a cultic scene, as the body is traditionally the locus of revelation and hierophany, while ritual knowledge is, some think, gained by and through the body (Grimes 1990).

The postsocialist milieu provided support for a strange, cultic environment of spiritualism and millennialism, which in turn strengthened spiritual affinity towards irrational, supernatural phenomena such as the activities of psychics, urban neoshamans and faith healers. Kürti (2001: 324) argues that the atmosphere of the post-totalitarian 'cultic age' expressing desires to negotiate between the sacred and the profane is one where, in millennial Hungary, 'mainstream and scientific ideas are blended with marginal and half-beliefs'. The Campbellian 'cultic milieu' in the postindustrial West and in the post-totalitarian East (Campbell 1972) shows the need for a re-enchantment of the world, as the disenchanted world of modernity no longer gives sufficient security (Beck 1992).

The postmodern syncretism of diverse medical realities is mirrored in the liminal state of the Hungarian medical system. Soon after the reorganisation of the Hungarian Chamber of Medicine in 1989 a dozen associations were founded for unconventional healers such as acupuncturists, homoeopaths, bioenergetists and Ayurvedic healers. The Hungarian Chamber of Alternative Medicine (*Természetgyógyászok Országos Kamarája*) was established in the early 1990s. Official surveys report a weak interest in unconventional medicine, while independent studies have uncovered a growing incidence of the use and acceptance of alternative medicine (Buda et al., this volume).

Partial transformation of the economic basis for treatment in certain strata of the medical system opened up new paths for enterprise in medicine. The increasing economic freedom induced innovations and the revival of traditional healing practices. Although the hegemony of biomedicine was not challenged at an institutional level during this period (on account of its evidence-based efficacy and use of high technology), extensive parallel use and acceptance of unconventional medicine – by 25 per cent of all patients – indicates the increasing legitimacy of 'alternative' attitudes regarding health (Buda et al., this volume). This interest is not simply a result of the transition, since one can find it in other historical periods, even during the last years of socialism, as proven by the interest in anti-cancer remedies such as Celladam or Béres Drops (Kürti 2001). The difference is that it became part of the structure only in the 1990s with the authorisation/legal regulation of complementary medicine.

This research is based on two years of multi-site fieldwork undertaken between 2001 and 2003 in Budapest. It was conducted among *táltos* healers and neoshamans whose activities I had been following since the mid-1990s (Lázár 1998). I focused on spiritual healing as a marginal field of unconventional medicine based on alternativist (spiritualist, animist or magico-religious) ontology. As these types of healing – in the context of associated rites of affliction – generate 'communitas' in a Turnerian sense among healers and patients, I tried to explore the role of embodiment of perceptions of non-ordinary reality in creating 'antistructure', as well as the dynamics of later reinstitutionalisation.

The medical system in plural transition

The stigmatisation of folk healers as fraudulent and ineffective, and the viewing of traditional popular medicine as a primitive and backward remnant of the magico-religious thinking of the past were common in the period of communist modernisation. These attitudes were general in the case of traditional healers in East-Central Europe and in the case of Siberian shamans whose mistreatment is described by Balzer (1999). Although the ideology of the class struggle slowly receded during the decades of 'socialism in reality', there was a period when these spiritualist or traditional healers represented a danger to the 'enlightened, scientific' dialectical materialist worldview and political system. They were victims of political persecution in the early 1950s and in the 1960s. For example, István Dóczi, a blind pastor, was one of those traditional healers labelled charlatans by officialdom; he was imprisoned several times in the 1950s and early 1960s (Gryneaus 2002).

The dismantling of the ideological hegemony of Marxism along with its exclusively materialist approach took place as result of the sociopolitical change-over in Hungary in 1989. This shift towards a monetarist free market postsocialism was accompanied by change in the medical system facilitating more free enterprise for those working outside hospitals, such as general practitioners and occupational health experts, as well as doctors 'emigrating' to the field of alternative medicine. In Hungary, sociopolitical transition created a comfortable space for the rapid evolution of alternative medicine. Transient legal tolerance opened paths for various forms of spiritual healing, too. On the other hand, legal regulation elevated the level of professionalism in the non-orthodox services, just as in other countries (Cant and Sharma 1999), and well-organised professional associations were formed to achieve control over the qualifications required. As a result of three pieces of legislation enacted in 1997, unconventional medicine has become a legitimate part of the healthcare system, a development that implied the integration of the antistructure created by unconventional medicine (COST B4 1998).

By Government Decree 40/1997(111.5) unconventional medicine became part of the healthcare system by *complementing* scientifically based medical practice. The 'rebuilt' structure expressing the social ranking and status hierarchy of the medical system is given by Order 11/1997 (V.28) of the Minister of Public Welfare (i.e., the minister for health) whereby it is for the medical doctor to govern diagnosis and therapy, while the practitioner of unconventional medicine is merely to complement the physician's activity, without countermanding or modifying his orders. The Order also identified those areas within unconventional medicine that can be practised and in which an officially recognised examination is possible. These fall into two groups. The first embraces activities to be carried out only by a medical doctor and includes homoeopathy, manual medicine, traditional Chinese medicine (TCM), Ayurvedic medicine, traditional Tibetan medicine, biological dentistry and anthroposophical medicine. Most of these healing practices – e.g., TCM, homoeopathy, Ayurvedic medicine and anthroposophical medicine – are based on spiritualist and non-materialist assumptions and include explanatory models dealing with Qi and meridians, subtle energy, prana, astral and mental body, and the philosophy of elements. The thinking underlying the legal regulation implied that healing based on unconventional ontology could merely complement the naturalist, positivist knowledge gained in the biomedicine curriculum.

The second group covers those activities practised without a MD degree, including acupressure, alternative gymnastics and massage, lifestyle therapy, reflexology, alternative physiotherapy, bioenergy, phytotherapy (herbalism) and kinesiology. Bioenergetics such as Touch for Health and healing through the laying on of hands constitute perhaps the most overlooked and astonishing revival of ancient and sacred healing practices, and, surprisingly, they do not require a biomedical background.

Medical sociological surveys (Buda et al., this volume) prove that in almost a quarter of patients neither religious constraints nor the influences of a materialistic educational background hinder the choice of acupuncture, bioenergy healing, acupressure, homoeopathy, chakra therapy or reiki. Although the non-materialistic content of such alternative healing practices is obvious, this content is usually not emphatic in the discourse regarding alternative healing. This is not surprising, since even in the case of religions the metaphysical background of the sacred is more or less muted. Modernist concepts of religion – based on Durkheim's (2003) assumption – conceive the sacred as simple projections of a social reality, where the sacred is ultimately the expression of social forces acting on the individual. As Gellner emphasises, in modernity most people take the canons of rationalism and science to be the only way of thinking, while relegating everything else to the informal sphere (Gellner 1974). In official discourse regarding alternative healing, the basic perceptions of alternative medicine as speculative, subjective, non-measurable by current scientific methods, hypothetical, spiritualistic and non-materialistic signify that these features and their given context are rather stigmatising. The idea of evidence-based complimentary medicine tells us 'the challenge is for therapies such as homoeopathy, hypnosis and anthroposophy to show they have a scientific base' (COST B4 1998: 13).

The field worker – like Janus – has two faces, one with an 'emic' smile and cultural relativist empathy tuned to cultural variance and one with a critical, 'etic' glance interested in universal explanations of phenomena. Embodied experience gained from healing rituals or walking on fire may offer transformative experience generating 'antistructure' not only for patients, but also for healers, and sometimes for anthropologists such as Goodman (1990) and Harner (Hoppál 1998), who may become members of the observed 'communitas' in a Turnerian sense. When a patient or a participant-observer experiences – in an altered state of consciousness or in other ways of embodying – strange or sacred sensations, he or she may be caught up in a different self-identification shared by the members of the ritual community. As Turner writes: 'Communitas, or social antistructure [is] a relational quality full of unmediated communication, even communion, between definite and determinate identities, which arises spontaneously in all kinds of groups, situations, and circumstances. It is a liminal phenomenon which combines the qualities of lowliness, sacredness, homogeneity, and comradeship' in contrast to ordinarily prevalent social structures (Turner and Turner 1978: 250). On the other hand, cultural relativism may protect against ritual joining of the antistructure. The particularist anthropological approach with its cultural relativist framework is not a science to reveal the truth in the background, but may help to bridge the gulf between knowledge gained from experiment and that gained from experience.

Cultural phenomenology of the body: the last station before the Transcendent

Mind and body cannot be isolated in kinesic practice, radiesthesia or other forms of embodiment considered as bodily ways of knowing. Csordas applies *embodiment* as a paradigm for anthropological understanding in the case of religious experiences, paranormal perceptions and personal experiences of unconventional healing. The self is seen as an integrated mind/body in reality inseparable from the social creation by which the subject is both generating and being generated (Csordas 1990). McGuire emphasises that social scientists must not isolate ideas from body practices, non-cognitive functions of the mind and the highly social aspects of mind/body/self, which require understanding of alternative definitions of reality and body itself (McGuire 1995). Diverse belief systems link the perceptual processes of healer and the patient with social constraints and cultural meanings through the body. This is why experience and not experiment, where (bodily) subjectivity must be excluded, is the source of knowledge in the case of alternative healing. The wide range of practices and experiences of alternative healing and the broad array of speculative ideologies regarding energies, subtle field, astral body, prana, chi, vis vitalis, od, PSI-energy and so forth create diverse mental realities which converge and turn out to be incompatible in some cases.

Without the 'hermeneutic shaping' of the bodily sensations of dowsing,[1] giving and receiving energy or feeling changes in astral space or subtle energy fields by way of the palm chakra, the actor cannot fill his internal and 'external' perceptions with meaning. The phenomenological approach helps to uncover the body as a sensor of hidden realities, the transfer of energies of unknown sources, or as the subject and object of total 'coenestopathic' transformation, such as becoming a power-animal: a fox or even a hawk. If alternative medicine can renew our experience regarding embodied consciousness, it will certainly offer material for phenomenological enquiry using the body as the crossroads of different consciousnesses. The final aim of the phenomenological reduction is to disclose the very essence *(eidé)* of the phenomena. Medical anthropological fieldwork helps us get close to the field of these bodily experiences. Bodily ways of knowing may be the common ground of very diverse fieldwork experiences, as in the case of bioenergetic healing based on dowsing, root shamanism and the postural induction of SSC (shamanic state of consciousness).

The *táltos* tradition and the postmodern Táltos

Contemporary Táltos[2] healers' practice is not really a continuation of the original *táltos* tradition, but rather a postmodern one, a sort of invention/reinvention of tradition. In the anthropological literature it was Kürti who first reported the Táltos activity (Kürti 2001). My fieldwork study, begun in the autumn of 2001, included one year's involvement as participant and observer in Táltos courses and, later on, interviewing, and gathering narratives from, various Táltos and neoshamanist healers.

To become a Táltos healer one has to attend weekend courses with ritualistic features. The enculturation includes alternativist, esoteric and spiritualist elements, as well as Hungarian ethno-cultural features. Videos with proofs of spiritual phenomena, walking on fire and dowsing (measuring geopathic radiation and sensing aura by radiesthesia) may be considered parts of an initiation rite, creating a new identity and conferring membership of a 'communitas' that offers transformation of the worldview and assists sharing in the counter-values of the Turnerian antistructure. The pronounced Magyar traditionalism involves learning traditional Hungarian *rovásírás* (runic writing), re-reading the legends of Hungarian saints royal and otherwise along with fairy tales with táltos contents, and occasional pilgrimages to sacred or cultic places, such as megalith remains in the Pilis or Bükk hill regions of Hungary. This spiritualist and esoteric praxis is mixed with Christian mysticism and with the cult of Christ and the Virgin Mary. The Táltos Church (*Táltos Egyház*), a new religion established in 1998, is one of the new ecclesiastical communities that emerged in the millennial cultic atmosphere (Kürti 2001). Táltos practice parallels the activity of similar alternativist healing centres in other countries, such as the ANAM Holistic Healing Center, which offers Celtic shamanism, shamanic healing, dowsing, divination workshops, and geopathic stress and land practices in Ireland, as well as guided tours of Celtic sacred sites, spiritual healing, and work to do with the aura, chakras and light body.

Táltos identity is expressed by elements of everyday wear, such as the *tarsoly* (a decorated bag worn on the belt). There are also educational materials, web pages, books, videos and journals published by the Táltos community. 'Communitas' values are reinforced through regular, informal meetings, the so-called Táltos *sala*. Postmodern syncretism is one of the most important features of contemporary Táltos healers, since they integrate almost every important branch of alternative healing – e.g., homoeopathy, acupressure, osteopathy, regressive hypnosis, bioenergetics, psychotronics and dowsing – with a pronounced ethnocultural identity, mystic Christianity and folklore. However, main symbols such as the Táltos drum show that these innovative efforts are from the emotional standpoint deeply anchored in the tradition.

Comparing the ancient *táltos* tradition and the newly invented Táltos practice the following (counter-)parallels can be drawn. In ethnic beliefs the *táltos*, similar to other superhuman beings in Hungarian folk beliefs such as the *garabonciás* (wizard able to raise storms), the *tudós* (man of knowledge) and the *látó* (seer), was thought to be marked out by a surplus finger given him by God in his mother's womb or by being born with '*táltos* teeth'. The *táltos* was elected by an initiatory vision: the *táltos* calling. The contemporary Táltos healer pays for the knowledge, although he is given the power through a laying on of hands by the leader, András Kovács. Other sources of the knowledge are thought to come from above, from angels or spirits as one of my informants, I. V., a 73-year-old retired worker, told me. It is interesting to note that the *javas* healer István Dóczi, mentioned above, received his knowledge from his grandfather by shaking hands with him, that the additional source of his knowledge was his archangel, and that he considered a *táltos* to be his protector.

The traditional *táltos* sorcerers distinguished themselves from witches, telling in their accounts that they healed people harmed by the witches 'not by diabolical skills or witchcraft but by virtue of godly science' (Klaniczay 1990: 138). My informants, Táltos healers of today, report successful faith healing of complaints caused by the evil eye, black magic and hexes. They heal by prayer, bringing the light on the sick person, sending energy or using other imaginative ways. The *táltos* in the past protected his community from evil forces and magical aggression; he fought for the fertility of the land, found the treasure in the land and influenced the weather. Nowadays Táltos healers are also thought to be able to find water or lost objects by dowsing.

The most striking shamanistic feature in the *táltos* tradition is *révülés* (the ecstatic capacity to fall into a trance). Contemporary Táltos healers are never in a real trance, but they induce in their patients a state of hypnosis, during which psychotronic surgery is performed using guided imagery. Dowsing, on the other hand, may be taken as a special form of an altered state of consciousness, one in which the person concerned remains fully alert and conscious. Táltos healers may make their diagnosis in a person's aura or, in the case of people not present, by using dowsing. In the case of auradiagnostics we can draw parallels with traditional *táltos* skills, such as Dóczi's divination-like diagnostics performed by 'scanning' the handkerchief of the patient using his fingers or a green stone given him by his grandfather, where the handkerchief serves as a map of the patient's body with representations of the patient's organs.

Led by the rod, healing by energy

The contemporary Táltos healers are representatives of an ancient way of healing well known all over the world (Brennan and Smith 1988, Targ and Katra 1998). This old healing tradition was a privileged and charismatic form of spiritual healing, one practised by the Apostles and royal saints. Distant psychic healing may be interpreted as 'a dynamic process that involves a field of persons and events – a field that is transspatial, transtemporal and transpersonal' (Braud, cited by Targ and Katra 1998: 219).

The transspatial and transtemporal medical reality of Táltos healers appears when a Táltos healer sends energy to a 'receiver' through an imagined mental 'phantom' of the given person in the case of long distance. The Táltos practice of healing by means of hands, meditation and prayer is more than unconventional: it is esoteric. Although healers in Táltos medicine have certification in unconventional medicine and official permission to practise reflexology, homoeopathy and chiropractics, Táltos clinical practice has predominantly esoteric and spiritual features, including psychotronics, faith healing and techniques for guided imagery.

The first step towards being a Táltos, becoming familiar with dowsing, may be interpreted as an esoteric initiation, making possible communication with the Inner Self or with information sources of unknown origin. Dowsing as a form of divination may be viewed as a cognitive embodied field of practical mastery used for healing, searching for things hidden from sight, seeking answers to questions, and directing appropriate conduct in critical situations (Tedlock 2001), or a means of talking with the divine or with the unconscious. Dowsing makes a person sensitive to geopathic radiation of several kinds thought to be pathogenic, and helps to scan the aura of others to reveal the signs of internal disease.

Dowsing is a real embodied process of gaining knowledge from 'outside and inside' at the same moment, or, as an old dowser once said, 'It is a window to the Almighty's will'. The first, initiatory, steps already help the Táltos healer to leave the world of materialist scepticism. When confronted with scientific, religious or commonsense denial of dowsing phenomena, dowsers feel growing commitment to the Turnerian 'communitas' with its antistructure character. The scientific denial of dowsing is based on the assertion that dowsing is not consistently repeatable and is an ideomotoric, subconscious activity governed indirectly by expectations rather than by conscious muscle activity. Both the religious and the scientific denial agree that dowsing is not consistent and may expose the dowser to ridicule, shame and failure, destroying all credibility. According to Hester, dowsing is thought to override our proven laws of physics and is positively destructive of our known reality (Hester 1984).

The perception of the hidden reality is not unequivocal to all actors by any means. The phenomenological approach offers a hermeneutical bypass to avoid the native's claim to 'positivist' evaluation of hidden realities, as well as to avoid scepticist denial of the hidden 'other world'. Results of dowsing are rarely replicable in controlled scientific studies; nevertheless a convergence of measurements was detectable among Táltos healer novices, and I observed the same thing among students of radiesthesia in the Biotér-Natura courses in dowsing, too. Embodied experience may be shaped or reconfigured socially during the teaching of these techniques of perception. It may be one of the 'body techniques' (Mauss 1935) used by the healers. Whether or not this convergence has a psychophysiological explanation on the basis of attribution-expectation or other unrevealed phenomena, here it is not our task to evaluate its relationship to 'commonsense reality'.

According to Táltos dowsers, the mind and body are indivisible in the gaining of information, since dowsing facilitates a sort of 'kinesiologic' communication with the unconscious, deeper self or the 'divine' part of the mind. From the cultural phenomenological point of view, dowsing by Táltos healers is based on socially informed embodiment of sensing 'changes in the astral world' and/or the 'environment of subtle energies'. Measuring geopathic lines, aura and chakras (seven energy centres along the body's axis) by dowsing exemplifies embodied knowledge expressing implicit, embodied and (sub-)culturally based practices. The changes measured by different dowsers are comparable. The common experience of making the invisible visible by dowsing – such as the locus in the aura of an actual disease, an anamnestic illness or the height of a distant person – may change our concept of space and time and even our concept of human being.

Invisible but touchable body as inverse avatar

As the occult diagnostician is enabled to diagnose the health status of a distant person by 'mind control' or by using a photograph, so the dowser may also test the 'phantom aura' of a distant person by using his rod. Like István Dóczi's handkerchief 'patient map', the auraphantom invoked and scanned by the Táltos healer may be seen as an esoteric counterpart of 'cyborgian simulated bodies', 'virtual cadavers' in cyberspace and virtual reality. Csordas (1997) gave a cultural phenomenological analysis of the virtual embodiment in cyberworld, when a person fitted out with the data gloves and data goggles involved in an advanced computerised simulation enters a virtual reality. When dowsing, the Táltos healer immerses himself in 'astral space' using his palm chakra, his 'astral glove'. While cyberspace is an intersubjective medium constituted socially (constituted by interaction among participants in the communicative medium), and virtual reality is the subjective sensory presence in that medium (constituted by interaction between individual user and technology), the dowsers' 'astral' reality is inside and outside social realities.

Simuloids, computer-generated humanoids and autonomous creatures are software-generated entities that have no sentient counterpart in actuality; they are software-controlled rather than human-controlled. Auraphantoms as objects of healing in the space 'scanable by dowsing' are inverse forms or counterparts of Avatars. As Csordas (1997) describes the cyber form of Avatars in cyberspace, the human computer operator may be analogous to a kind of deity that manipulates the computerised Avatar in virtual human form. The 'astralphantom' diagnosed by a dowser is just the opposite, an invisible empty space, where the (pre-objective?) embodied sensation of a distant person's bodily changes is disclosed by the bodily changes of the dowser, made visible by the rod for conscious analysis. Using the rod, most dowsers, acting independently of one another, select the same place for geopathic radiation, the same height of a person, and the same locus of a patient's illness. The other person is represented by embodied sensations, but it is the community of Táltos dowsers that shapes these perceptions.

The invisible explored by radiesthesia is filled with meaning. As a 27-year-old Táltos novice working as a computer engineer told me:

> I was frustrated with materialism, I lacked the larger part of the world, and when I started to sense the hidden reality, I felt as a patient is wont to feel after an operation on his eyes, when the bandages are taken off. Or when somebody opens both eyes and starts to perceive spatial relations instead of a simple, two-dimensional picture.

These unconventional experiences create a different perception of hidden realities, as the embodied perception of the other person made visible by the dowser rod creates cultural reality for the Táltos healers and for other dowsers, too. It may change the pragmatic aspects of medical wisdom, as a medical doctor, a 36-year-old public health expert, practising dowsing says:

> *Gnoti se auton.* One may know his real entity. It is revealing. But one gets to know the real limitations, too. Dowsing let me reveal the extent of the role of patients in their healing, since without their volition, participation and asking we can achieve nothing. I learned the limitations of empathy also. For me it is a great gift to experience limitlessness in space and time, but I have to confront a more serious uncertainty regarding what really happened. One can liberate the serious cancer patient from the predestining judgment of statistics; the doors of fate can be opened by trust and faith.
>
> I gained pragmatic belief based on personal experience, or, one can say, personal experience of miracles instead of the good old formal, conventional beliefs. Wisdom instead of calculative rationality.

As dowsing itself is thought to be a form of initiation, some dowsers create real antistructure framework when applying dowsing to healing (they do this without payment, strictly on request and in teams where they may check each other's results). Since Táltos healers have a clinical framework for healing and their practice is mixed with homoeopathy, this antistructure framework is not obvious in a clinical setting. More spiritualistic dowsers sometimes criticise the people selling these exceptional healing capabilities.

The non-ordinary reality of Táltos healing

The greatest risk in unconventional healing is to substitute and block a more effective biomedical remedy for a serious illness. Patients who consider – often erroneously – their neoplastic disease incurable may eschew oncological care and turn to alternative healers. Such behaviour may prove fatal if, for example, somebody has a mammary carcinoma or other neoplasm that is curable provided that the therapy is given early enough. This is why academic experts reject bioenergetic or other unconventional healing for serious diseases (Makó 1998). Regarding the scientific reality of the subtle energies and aura, the need for debate is obvious (Rasmussen 1995), but the 'social reality' of these targets of healing is unquestionable.

Here we offer an example of Táltos healing of a neoplasm judged inoperable by a neurosurgeon. We have abundant data on the self-limited growth of tumours, and the case study is not evaluable from the biomedical point of view, as we do not know the histology, the malign or benign nature of the tumour. Nevertheless it is worth discussing because 'mental surgery' is perhaps the most radical alternativist method in the Táltos healing 'arsenal', depicting the practical dimension of this spiritual ontology, illustrating the use of an altered state of consciousness and showing the ritual elements of Táltos healing.

Mrs Lajos Péli, a 70-year-old retired teacher, had been repeatedly hospitalised because of fluctuating neurological symptoms, vomiting, dysphagy, confused speech and progressive paralysis of the right side of her body that developed in February and March 2002. Following the accurate diagnosis of a neoplasm (2.0 x 1.0 x 1.5 cm in size) with perifocal oedema infiltrating the pons and the cerebellum made via CT and MRI scans by medical staff, and following a consultation with a neurosurgeon, pharmacological treatment was chosen to reduce the oedema around the tumour. The surgical intervention had a high risk to benefit ratio, and neither irradiation, nor chemotherapy was suggested, although a glycerol, steroid therapy was started to slow down the progress of paralysis. The family turned to the Táltos Clinic for alternative medical help on their own initiative. As the serious physical condition and paralysis of the patient made her hardly movable, a Táltos healer, Imre Kercselics, offered a 'spirit surgery' intervention with the help of the patient's son. The son – an academic expert in the social sciences working abroad – travelled home to join the unconventional healing process. Spirit surgery means an imaginary surgery by which the tumour is eradicated at the level of the patient's spirit, in the hope that this will be transcribed to the material level should the participants have sufficiently strong belief. Similar spirit surgery operations have been made by Vilmos Csontos in Zseliz, Slovakia, and a similar syncretist healing that fuses Afro-Brazilian folk religion and ideas drawn from medical science is reported in Porto Alegre (Greenfield 1992).

'Spirit surgery' implies religious and magical elements, prayer, meditation and symbolic operation in a state of trance. Spirit surgery of this kind enables the closest blood relatives (son, brother, parents) to help by acting on the patient's spiritual and material body via imaginative methods guided by the spirit surgeon. In this spiritual healing ritual the son of the patient passed through a sort of initiation needed for effective participation. He described the clinical milieu and the process:

The patients sitting around were ordinary people, nothing special. Even the healer was a simple, average man. But the clinical environment decorated with spiritual paintings and carved wooden sculptures was very impressive. I was given a cassette to learn the sequential process of imagination. During the healing act I soon became relaxed, and during the guided imagery I went down 21 steps; I had to drink from the water of life, eat a leaf from the tree of life, and with a winged white 'táltos' horse we flew up to the heavenly castle of the Lord, where I asked forgiveness. I was given a sword, white coat and helmet from the Lord. Then we went to the spirit hospital, where the 'virtual' operation on the tumour was completed. It is important to mention that after the spiritual operation, for weeks I had to send energy in an altered state of consciousness, getting down the stairway, drinking from the spring of water of life ten times and sending the energy, and repeating a formula: 'I trust in my mother's spirit, that it will heal my mother's body 100 per cent.'

He was participating seriously in the healing process and became a member of the antistructure; nevertheless he could keep his distance and find his way back.

Basically I don't feel that it changed my worldview, as I was open to the transcendental and I somehow always believed in these things. Simply, just following a Popperian physicist orientation – extending the concept of the material world, as was not infrequent in the history of physics – I thought that acupuncture, acupressure and other alternative healing methods were just as natural as electricity and magnetism previously woven into the net of rationality. It is interesting that I did not want to decide what was true. Unbelievable events used to make me sceptical, but I now think that things have multiple 'readings'. In the case of alternative healings one cannot find causal relationships, but the beneficial outcomes may become more frequent.

The mother deepened her religious spiritualism, experiencing rapid improvement after the therapy and complete remission during the next three weeks. While her son was sending the energy, she sometimes perceived sudden feelings of warmth, which she attributed to her son only later on.

After the spiritual healing I started to pray and forgive everybody. It was a marvellous feeling. I had a conventional faith before and this experience caused me to be more spiritual. I felt a sort of metanoia.

Her paralysis was resolved and she is free from any symptoms two years after the diagnosis. As she was taking glycerol and corticosteroid to reduce the oedema around the tumour, this therapy was rather an example of a mixed treatment of a neoplasm, so the remission can be rationalised on the basis of different models such as biomedical neurological or psycho-immunological explanations too.

'Outbodiment' or visiting the spirits' world

Experiencing fields of subtle energy, astral space and aura by dowsing is almost like entering a discovered world, without leaving one's own. 'Dasein'[3] is not questioned; one is alert, and can measure, test, compare, conclude and behave rationally based on an embodied experience of the hidden. The healer is alert when 'talking' with his unconscious, and perceives only the motion of an unquiet dowsing rod, or subtle internal bodily changes. In neoshamanic healing it is not the healer but the patient who sinks into an altered state of consciousness (ASC) to sense different realities.

At Jonathan Horwitz's shaman course in Budapest in the late 1980s, Gábor Elekes and his colleagues acquainted themselves with the technique of the 'shamanic journey' in practice. They were influenced by Istvan Somogyi, leader of the Arvisura Theatre, whose neoshamanistic activity is reported in Kürti's article on the Cultic Milieu in Hungary (Kürti 2001). The structure of a continually working shaman drumming group in a psychiatric ward took shape in those sessions held at the Cserkút Centre. Here we can find contact between cultic counter-culture and an experimental medical sub-culture. With Jungian depth psychology as the theoretical background, Gábor Elekes, a clinical psychologist on the Children's and Young People's Psychiatric Ward at Szolnok Hospital, started to help youngsters between the ages of thirteen and eighteen years by applying some parts of shamanic work. This 'radical shamanistic' experience became part of the official psychiatric healing work applied by two creative psychologists, Orsolya Czaga and Gábor Elekes, from the late 1990s onwards.

Their group at the National Psychiatric and Neurological Institute operated for three years, from 1998 until 2001; they continued to use techniques of shamanic healing in psychiatric work in outpatient care there and, more recently, in a drumming group on the psychiatric ward of Kistarcsa's Ferenc Flór Hospital among mainly schizophrenic patients, addicts and depressed patients. Orsolya Czaga told about the ritual content of their method in August 2002 in an interview:

> The group was started as an experiment, for as far as we know, shamanic rituals have never been used in academic psychiatric therapy. Our group uses the approach and rituals of the shamanic religion, but these are interpreted as psychological functions in our method.

The techniques applied consist of shamanic rituals with drums, rattles, song and dance, with verbal, pictorial and group talks to integrate the experience. Resistance to therapy for religious reasons is not infrequent, but Orsolya tells:

> I can say that to practise shamanism it's not necessary to believe in it. What is necessary? It is the way in which the spiritual experience becomes a reality in one's own life.

Six to eight patients take part in a session. The rituality structures the time; controls social relations, communication and behaviour; and offers security in the exaggerated liminality infringing the borders of different realities. As a framework, at the beginning and end of a session the participants sit in a circle and hold each other's hands, an action that *takes them out of profane space and time* and produces group-cohesion. This 'communitas' offers a transient membership of antistructure playing a role in the healing of the Self. Rattling helps to prepare the imaginative way for communication with the 'helper spirits'. From the view of psychology, spirit-helpers can be regarded as expressive symbols of different aspects of the personal and collective unconscious. In the ritual the patients give voice to imagined helper animals, and this way they may invoke the supportive impulses of the sphere of instincts regarding the Jungian explanatory model used by Czaga and Elekes. Rattling and drumming, dance and singing help the patients' personal and 'cultural regression'.

There is a crucial difference between clinical neoshamanism and the classic shamanistic rituals, just as there are differences between shamanism and altered states of consciousness in Leuner's KB[4] (Lázár 1993). Here it is not the shaman – in the present case the psychologist – but the patient who makes a journey accompanied by drumbeat. This happens in a relaxed position for about twenty minutes. The patient makes a journey with the help of drumbeat into the Lower, Middle and Upper World of non-ordinary reality, each expressing different types of problem solving.

During the neoshamanistic healing rite the patients work in pairs, too. One is in a passive relaxed state open to the alternate reality. The other person plays the role of healer, diagnosing positive fields on his partner's body. His experience is described using shamanic terminology: As Orsolya tells:

> He is helped by his rattle and helpers, who are 'called' before the journey. When he feels their presence, he kneels down beside the patient. He raises his hands above the patient's body, and when the rattle signals by changing its sound, or when the healer can feel something special with the palm of his hand (e.g., a change in the temperature, a stitch or stiffening), he closes his eyes and tries to see the non-ordinary image of that field.

These words depict the embodiment of the non-ordinary reality, which parallels subtle perceptions during sensing of the aura.

After the drumbeat has called the participants back from their journey, they put down their experiences in notes. The retrospective descriptions, drawings and paintings of the 'primitive reality' experienced helps to catalyse the therapeutic change. The patients share their experience with the group. One aim of the therapy is to build the information obtained into the participant's real life.

The parallel terminologies (*the language of shamanism, depth psychology* and *everyday language*) indicate that healers and patients may experience multiple medical realities even in one therapy (neoshamanistic, Jungian and aspecific group therapy contexts). This multiplicity may help to overcome religious resentments toward neoshamanistic therapy, and (neo)shamanistic therapy may also become acceptable for those who appreciate only scientific approaches. The healers' professional careers show how the shamanistic tradition may again reach mainstream medicine by way of the chain of antistructure transformations. Jung created the antistructure in the Freudian psychoanalytic social structure through his rebellious ideas, while Harner, Horwitz and Goodman – transforming the phenomena observed into action – created an antistructure by their neoshamanistic practice in the world of anthropology. These changes helped our psychologists in the transformation of neoshamanistic counter-culture antistructure into the experimental practice of mainstream psychiatry.

The body opens up the past

Felicitas Goodman's archaeological anthropology, or, as she calls it, psychological archaeology, takes us further back in the past. Here the body is not a vehicle for the soul or spirits; rather it is the bodily posture that shapes the way to the hidden reality. Goodman's anthropological discovery – with re-enchanting anthropology itself – challenged the functionalist anthropological audience, as she reports in her book (Goodman 1990). She and her co-workers investigated trance states induced by gestures and postural patterns preserved by Neolithic sculptures and figures. She discovered more than thirty positions inducing trance states with different specific sensations and visions but with the same ·electrophysiological mental state. We verified the same electrophysiological features of enhanced interoception with right hemispherical shift of alpha electroencephalographic (EEG) activities in trance induction in hypnosis and progressive relaxation (Lázár and Papp 1990).

In April 1993 Felicitas Goodman organised a one-week course with the participation of 120 people in three groups. During this week eight postural trances – classified as healing, mantic, energiser, traveller and mythopoetic trances – were taught. As the leader of the group, Pál Fuferenda, a teacher aged forty-six, explained the embodied sensation of those subtle changes caused by postural trance induction was enough to convince most of the participants of the existence of spiritual reality. In these sessions rattles were used for acoustic stimulation, and the sessions lasted for fifteen minutes. The chosen posture and the breathing exercises helped participants to reach a peculiar trance state specific to every postural type. Pál Fuferenda mentioned the four different clusters of postures – metamorphic, energiser, healing and mantic – used most frequently. In a metamorphic induction, for example, participants may sometimes experience coenestopathic, embodied feeling of being animals, or other beings. As his power-animal was a fox, in the trance state he felt that he had a long red tail:

I felt my hair growing, touching my shoulders. Looking back I realised that I had a red tail. I realised I was a fox, and not a human being, surrounded by little foxes, children of mine. For a little while I tried to imagine how my family members and colleagues would accept these changes. But soon I was immersed in the new situation, I became my power-animal, the Fox.

Most of the participants of the groups remained active, carrying on the research regarding postural trances and completing the list of trance-inducing postures with a further twenty positions. Later they organised the so-called Open Worlds Foundation providing a framework for the publication of books and the teaching of the method to others. Although these experimental trance states were sought out as a special hermeneutic device for obtaining more information about religions and rituals of the past, they became a source of the neoshamanic rituals of the present. The experimental practice of postural trance was converted into a therapeutic method applied among thirty to fourty drug addicts in 1997 and 1998 and used together with NADA[5] ear acupuncture treatment at Szentendre Holistic House. They offered shamanic state of consciousness as a 'drug-free journey', as a competitive blocker of hunger for drugs.

Some of the experimental group and those gathering at the Szentendre Holistic House in 2001 formed a new religious community, calling themselves 'Children of the Light, Hungarian Essenic Church', extending their interest towards Reiki as represented by Strohm.

Conclusions

In the Hungary of the post-totalitarian transition we can find a *mixed medical system* involving alternative fields of healing open to a wide range of medical traditions and rich in the healing cults integrating shamanism and esoterism. We focused on the revival of shamanism as a resurgence of the most ancient form of healing. Shamanism may be handled as a healing paradigm for complementary therapy (Money 2001) and, through the embodied perceptions of non-ordinary reality gained by an altered state of consciousness, this healing practice may offer a ritualised transformative experience for the participants.

We could describe the transformative consequences of experience gained from neoshamanist procedures, not only at the individual but also at the microsocial level, using Turner's structure/'communitas' model. This experience is not only embodied, but may work on the social body generating antistructure, or counter-culture institutions, alternative clinics, Holistic Health centres, Táltos schools, or newly established small churches. This generating force can be explained not only by economical reasons: the embodied experience of non-ordinary reality may be one of the most dynamic sources of its 'social energy'.

The other way of returning to structure from 'communitas' is the latter's reintegration into mainstream medical practice. If there are translators and mediators who are well equipped to explain and utilise explanatory models, such as our psychologists with their Jungian depth psychological background, they can open the doors closed by ideological 'gatekeeper' mechanisms. The example of the drumming group practice followed since Horwitz's neoshamanistic training to the renewed healing canons of the psychiatric ward proves this possibility.

The exchange of explanatory models gained from different healing practices may even modify the basic concepts of health and illness, just as it may the basic view of a human being as a pure biological system, spiritual entity or energetic being. This embodied knowledge needs further evaluation via a renewed methodology of cooperative enquiry based on a participatory worldview extending our approach to the unified analysis of experiential, presentational, propositional and practical knowing and their interactions in unconventional healing (Heron 2001).

What these unconventional therapies offer by their rituals to those dismembered by frustration and illness is no less than to re-member them into their new 'communitas' and remember the miracles of an enchanted world. The 'disenchanted' clockwork nature of modernity obeys mechanistic natural laws rather than spiritual ones. The spiritual experiences of certain healing practices repopulate this clockwork with the hidden dynameia of the supernatural. In the cases of helpless states of chronic debilitating diseases and incurable cancers, mechanistic, predictable nature brings bad news for both patient and healer. While the body remains a 'thing', it is constrained by the power of the statistical laws of a mechanistic world, but if the person as a sacred, unique being frees himself from statistical determinations, the world of miracles is opened up, at least in his mind.

Notes

1. Dowsing is the action of a person – called a dowser – using a rod, stick or other device. Dowsing emphasises special small movements in the hand using a movable device, rod or pendulum. Since dowsing is not based upon any known scientific or empirical laws or forces of nature, it should be considered a type of divination.
2. The Táltos healer as representative of a postmodern syncretist unconventional healing sub-culture is signified by the use of a capital T to distinguish him or her from the *táltos* tradition in folklore heritage, a tradition denoted by the use of italics all in the lower case.
3. A Heideggerian term for 'being-there', the kind of existence that self conscious human beings uniquely possess.
4. In the so called Leuner 'Katathym Bilderleben'-technique or guided affective imagery one experiences an altered state of consciousness through relaxation followed by mental imagery. The archetypic images that appear during the 'mental journey' may mimic a trip in an alternative reality. After returning to normal awareness the therapist initiates a discussion in order to identify a series of motifs, all with specific symbolic psychodynamic meaning, to be evoked and elaborated in the therapeutic session.

5. NADA is short for the 'National Acupuncture Detoxicification Association', who since the 1980s has developed a five point acupuncture programme for detoxification after abuse of alcohol or drugs

References

Balzer, M.M. 1999. *The Tenacity of Ethnicity: A Siberian Saga in Global Perspective.* Princeton: Princeton University Press.

Beck, U. 1992. *Risk Society: Towards a New Modernity.* London: Sage.

Brennan, B. 1988. *Hands of Light: Guide to Healing Through the Human Energy Field.* New York: Bantam Books.

Campbell, C. 1972. The Cult, the Cultic Milieu and Secularization, in Hill, M. (ed.) *A Sociological Yearbook in Britain.* London: SCM Press.

Cant, S. and U. Sharma. 1999. *A New Medical Pluralism.* London: Routledge.

COST B4. 1998. *Unconventional Medicine. Final Report of the Management Committee 1993–1998.* Luxembourg: The European Commission.

Csordas T.J. 1990. 'Embodiment as a Paradigm for Anthropology', *Ethos* 18: 5–47.

——1997. *'Computerized Cadavers: Shades of Being and Representation in Virtual Reality.'* Paper to the Conference 'After Post-Modernism'. http://www.focusing.org/apm_papers/compucad.html

Durkheim E. 2003 (1912). *A vallási élet elemi formái* [The Elementary Forms of Religious Life]. Budapest: L'Harmattan Kiadó.

Gellner, E. 1974. *Legitimation of Belief.* Cambridge: Cambridge University Press.

Goodman, F.D. 1990. *Where the Spirits Ride the Winds.* Bloomington Indianapolis: Indiana University Press.

Greenfield, S.M. 1992. 'Spirits and Spiritist Therapy in Southern Brazil: a Case Study of an Innovative, Syncretic Healing Group', *Culture, Medicine and Psychiatry* 16: 23–51.

Grimes, R.L. 1990. *Ritual Criticism: Case Studies in its Practice, Essays on its Theory.* Columbia S.C.: University of South Carolina Press.

Grynaeus T. 2002. *A fehértói javas ember tudománya* [Knowledge of the 'javas' healer from Fehértó]. Szeged: Csongrád Megyei Könyvtári Füzetek.

Heron, J. 2001. 'The Placebo Effect and a Participatory World View', in D. Peters (ed.) *Understanding the Placebo Effect in Complementary Medicine.* London: Churchill, Livingstone.

Hester, B. 1984. *Dowsing,* http://www.sdanet.org/atissue/books/dowsing/index.htm

Hoppál, M. 1998. 'Urban Shamans: a Cultural Revival', in A.-L. Siikala and M. Hoppál (eds) *Studies on Shamanism.* Helsinki: Finnish Anthropological Society, 197–209.

Klaniczay, G. 1990. *The Uses of Supernatural Power.* Cambridge: Polity Press.

Kopp, M. 2000. 'Cultural Transition', in G. Fink (ed.) *The Encyclopedia of Stress.* New York: Academic Press.

Kürti, L. 2001. 'Psychic Phenomena, Neoshamanism and the Cultic Milieu in Hungary', *Nova Religio* 4(2): 322–351.

Lázár, I. 1993. 'Common Features of the Shamanic Trance and the Altered State of Consciousness in Leuner's KB (Katathym Bilderleben)', paper to the International Conference on Shamanism and Performing Arts, July 14 1993, Budapest.

——1998. 'Léleknyomon' Orvosi antropológiai széljegyzet [Tracing the Soul Medical Anthropological Notes on the Margin], *Komplementer Medicina* (Budapest) 7: 26.

Lázár, I. and Z. Papp. 1990. 'Simultaneous Thermography and Brain Mapping in Altered States of Consciousness', paper at the 'Vth International Congress of Psychophysiology', July 2 1990, Budapest.

Makó, J. (1998) 'Látlelet a természetgyógyászatról' [Diagnosis of Unconventional Medicine], *Természet Világa* 129: 10.

Mauss M. 1973 (1935). 'Techniques of the Body' (Translated by B. Brewster), *Economy and Society* 2(1): 70–87.

McGuire, M. 1995. 'Alternative Therapies: The Meaning of Bodies in Knowledge and Practice', in H. Johannessen, S.G. Olesen and J. Andersen (eds) *Studies in Alternative Therapy 2, Body and Nature*. Odense: INRAT and Odense University Press, 15–32.

Money M.C. 2001. 'Shamanism as a Healing Paradigm for Complementary Therapy', *Complementary Therapies in Nursing & Midwifery* 7: 126–31.

Rasmussen, I.L. 1995. 'Energies of the Body?', in H. Johannessen, S.G. Olesen and J. Andersen (eds) *Studies in Alternative Therapy 2, Body and Nature*. Odense: INRAT and Odense University Press, 136–145.

Schopflin, G. 2002. 'New-old Hungary: A Contested Transformation', *East European Perspectives* 4(10): http://www.rferl.org/eepreport/

Targ R. and J. Katra. 1998. *Miracles of Mind: Exploring Non-local Consciousness and Spiritual Healing*. New York: New World Library.

Tedlock, B. 2001. 'Divination as a Way of Knowing: Embodiment, Visualization, Narrative and Interpretation', *Folklore* 112(2): 189–197.

Turner, V. 1982 'Social Dramas and Stories About Them' in V. Turner, *From Ritual to Theatre: The Human Seriousness of Play*. New York: PAJP, 61–88.

Turner, V. and E. Turner. 1978. *Image and Pilgrimage in Christian Culture*. New York: Columbia University Press.

4

'The Double Face of Subjectivity'
A Case Study in a Psychiatric Hospital (Ghana)

Kristine Krause

Sickness requires us to acknowledge the double face of subjectivity, for people are subjects in relation to affliction, in that they form ideas about it and act upon it, and they are also subject to it as it strikes them down and sometimes resists their attempts to manage it. They undergo and undertake (Whyte 2002: 172).

The 'double face of subjectivity', aptly summarised by Susan Reynolds Whyte, as undergoing and undertaking, points to one of the major challenges of Medical Anthropology: How to bring together perspectives of sociopolitical structures and power relations with perspectives of suffering, recovering and acting subjects (Johannessen, this volume). On the one hand, one needs to shed light on the processes by which subjects and objects of medical practices are constituted and medical knowledge is authorised. On the other hand, it is necessary to develop analytical tools which are capable of grasping the sometimes inconsistent acts of the people involved.[1] Concerning this challenge Michael Lambek states: 'Agency is a tricky concept. Leave it out and you have a determinist or abstract model, put it in and you risk instrumentalism, the bourgeois subject, the idealised idealistic individual etc. But we can see how agents are always partly constructed through their acts – constituted through acts of acknowledgement, witnessing, engagement, commitment, refusal and consent' (Lambek 2002: 37).

In this paper I try to reconstruct those 'acts of acknowledgement, refusal and consent' in a state-owned psychiatric hospital in Ghana.[2] First, I am going to show how members of the staff combine biomedical treatment with Christian healing and, then, how this specific offer is appropriated by a female patient.[3] Biomedical care is the predominant treatment in this hospital.

However, in the practice of the Christian group, whose members are mostly biomedically trained and whose leader was the leading psychiatrist of the clinic at the time of my research, one finds two intertwined ways of treatment that construe the sickness of patients in different but complementary ways. From a historical perspective the Christian and the biomedical discourse appear paradigmatically incompatible in the sense that the development of modern psychiatry was heralded when the notion that spirits cause disease was abandoned (Foucault 1972 [1961], Gordon 1988: 24). As the paper is going to illustrate, the competition for competence in the Ghanaian context is not so much between science and religion but between different religious practices. After sketching the medical and religious scene in Ghana, I present in the first part of the paper the specific practices of the Christian group in using the concept of structural affinity outlined by Helle Johannessen in the introduction to this volume. In the second part I analyse the narration of one female patient in order to show how, on the one hand, she is partly in consent with it yet, on the other hand, refuses to subject herself totally to the Christian and biomedical discourse. To do so, I first note a few thoughts on the 'double face of subjectivity' to sketch a theoretical frame in which to analyse my material.

Subjunctive aspects in acts of appropriation

The difficulty to reconstruct agency and agents as mentioned in the beginning becomes more evident in the context of a psychiatric institution. As Michel Foucault has pointed out the historical formation of psychiatry and institutions like prisons and modern citizenship demarcated the reasonable and intelligible subject in contrast to the abject other (Rose 1992b, Butler 1993: reference 4, Foucault 1972 [1961]). Thus it seems paradoxical to look for the acting subjects in an institution which relies on concepts and practices of mental disorder that by interdiction negate the agency and citizenship qualities of the patients. Yet Nikolas Rose, following Foucault, analyses in his work how the assumed contradiction between subjectivity and power disguises the relations by which power works *through* and not *against* subjectivity (Rose 1992a: 142ff). In a recent volume on 'Postcolonial Encounters' edited by Richard Werbner (2002), several authors, Susan Reynolds Whyte among them, took up the task of rethinking subjectivity and agency. Werbner defines subjectivity in three dimensions: as *political* (subjugation under authorities like the state), as *moral* (rights and duties which are burdened on the subject), and as *existential* (personal and intimate relations) (Werbner 2002: 2). In her contribution Whyte offers the term *subjunctivity* to describe how 'the situated concerns' of people are dealt with and how justice could be done to the 'double face of subjectivity'.[4]

In my opinion the term opens up a way of thinking about how, in processes of subjugation to *body politics* (Lock and Schepher-Hughes 1996:

61ff, Johannessen, this volume), moments of resistance and reinterpretation are articulated by appropriating medical or religious discourses aiming at solutions for specific problems. Grammatically speaking, subjunctivity fits between indicative and imperative as the mood of a verb to express conditions and possibilities. It is therefore the way in which we express our concerns and hopes and take possession of given interpretations of the world. Transferred to the field of social practices, subjunctivity marks the existential moment where the undergoing meets the undertaking, although not as the heroic action of a single subject but more like idiosyncratic aspects emerging in specific interactive situations that in a medical setting are structured by ruling patterns of diagnosis and treatment procedures.

My argument here is that in order to recognise aspects of agency within the articulation of people who are considered to be mad, we have to grasp the subjunctive aspects: that is, the aspects where people try to act and give meaning to conditions *through* their entanglements and not against them. In my opinion we could find these subjunctive aspects by carefully considering their acts of *appropriating*[5] the given discourses. The focus on appropriation strategies – articulations through and not against subjugation – might help us further to explain how pluralistic medical practices are socially realised. Its relevance is therefore not restricted to 'oddnography'[6] but to ethnography as well.

The analysis of appropriations in this paper is twofold. First, I elaborate on the absorption and transformation of the biomedical discourse by a specific Christian Charismatic belief system, and second how this syncretistic medical practice is then again appropriated by a patient in a subjective way. Following the patient's interpretation of her sickness I illustrate how she, in her dealings with the spirits disturbing her, interprets social conflicts. This, I argue, enables her to come to her own terms with the diagnosis that categorises her sickness as 'chronic schizophrenia' (biomedical diagnosis) and the spirits possessing her as 'agents of the devil' (Christian diagnosis).

Medical and religious pluralism

As Whyte observed, since the 1970s a shift has occurred in the research on religious and medical practices in Africa from 'religion to medicine' (Whyte 1989). During the same time period the World Health Organisation (WHO) aimed to support in a programmatic way the cooperation with so-called traditional healers at the primary healthcare level.[7] The spiritual aspects of traditional medicine, however, cannot simply be standardised, and have thereby eluded the evaluation criteria of the WHO, which follow the biomedical paradigm, mostly focusing on herbal medicine (Ventevogel 1996: 4ff). Yet precisely these elusive aspects contribute, among other things, to the popularity of the alternate healing methods offered. Biomedicine cannot explain *why* a particular disease strikes this or that person. By contrast, the social and moral dimensions of an affliction that could provide answers to such questions are discussed in the 'social causation theories' of the traditional healers, as Twumasi states for Ghana (Twumasi 1979: 349).

One cannot speak of adequate biomedical psychiatric care for the population in Ghana, a country with only three psychiatric clinics.[8] However, we do find a variety of medical practices within the medical set up of Ghanaian society. People take up extensively the treatments offered by various healers (Twumasi 1975: 9ff, Osei 1997: 132f). Sometimes practitioners distinguish themselves from others by using mutually exclusive categories like religious/nonreligious and natural/supernatural, Christian/non-Christian, modern/traditional. The drawing of such strict disciplinary boundaries needs to be understood as a political and economic strategy in the publicly contested medical field in Ghana. We find herbalists, bonesetters, traditional midwives, muslim healers like mallams and marabouts, possession priests like *trŏnua* among the Ewe, *akomfo* among the Akan, Tigare and Mami Wata Shrines and a variety of Christian healers and prophets.[9] However, the different methods are not neutral vis-à-vis one another. A social and cultural ranking of medical practices as well as competition and supportive networking can be observed. One of the results of longstanding research in medical pluralism in Africa is that the health-seeking behaviour of the people is much more guided by pragmatic decisions and personal networks in the therapy-managing group, than in decisions for or against the underlying principles of one medical system. This applies for the Ghanaian case as well (Mullings 1984, Fink 1987, Ventevogel 1996).

The activities of the Christian Charismatic group in the clinic are therefore to be seen in the context of inadequate biomedical care facilities, on the one hand, and the countless offerings of various healers competing with each other, on the other. In turn, the Charismatic Christians – who themselves belong to this alternative scene – demonise all the other healing methods for being in their eyes, among other things, the very source of sickness themselves.[10] Therefore any attempt to include alternate methods of treatment at the primary healthcare level in Ghana – which is still on the agenda of the Ministry of Health (Osei 1999) – does face serious difficulties: medical pluralism in Ghana needs to be seen as religious pluralism, too. In this context, the therapeutic practice of the Fellowship in the clinic fills a void; to a certain extent it replaces the utter lack of psychotherapeutic care, for in the clinic the patients are just 'kept in custodial care' and 'only' treated with medicines.

In the introduction to this volume, Helle Johannessen proposed to conceptualise medical pluralism not as the coexistence of separate and independent sociocultural systems of medicine, but as networks based on affinal organising principles. This perspective goes beyond the assumed incompatibility of, for example, biomedical treatment and religious healing. It provides a useful framework for analysing the practices in the psychiatric clinic.

The members of the Christian Fellowship who prescribe biomedical drugs and 'anointing prayers' at the same time are not only biomedical experts but also ritual experts in the arts of Christian Charismatic healing. This leads to the following question: how do the members of the fellowship combine the two practices and ideologies in their daily routine, and how are relations of affinity created?

Relations of affinity in biomedical treatment and Christian healing

Both healing methods used by the Christian Fellowship in the hospital claim universal authorities for themselves: those of the natural sciences and those of the Holy Spirit. As in other biomedical subdisciplines, standards for biomedical psychiatry are set by the World Health Organization (WHO). The WHO claims global authority in defining sickness and health and offers standardised and internationally recognised education and diagnostic manuals like the ICD-10, which are used in the Ghanaian clinics as well (Kleinman 1995, chapter 2, Wolf and Stürzer 1996: VIII). Charismatic Christianity – as with other streams in Christianity – claims to possess the true understanding of the Bible and ritual practices. In order to assert this claim, its adherents refer to its spread on a global scale. This spread is visible in the global spiritual warfare as well as in the actual networks of support, which have been established by Charismatic churches. Charismatic Christianity – also known as the Revivalist or 'Born-Again' Neo-Pentecostal movement – has meanwhile become the fastest growing Christian denomination worldwide. It is very successful in areas that have been subject to rapid transformations and exhibit an extreme polarisation of wealth and poverty, such as Africa, Latin America, but also in the Pacific region and in South Korea.[11]

The ritual practices of Charismatic Christians refer to a belief system whose core consists of the 'gifts of the Holy Spirit' which enabled Christ's Apostles to perform miracles as Jesus himself did.[12] Among these wondrous deeds are the healing of diseases, the gift of prophecy, teaching and preaching as well as the gift of speaking in tongues. The Christian Fellowship in the clinic was founded 1996 by the senior psychiatrist Dr Kanyi*.[13] Ten to fifteen clinical staff members form the core group. A prayer is offered once a week that includes ritual elements like drumming, dancing, singing, speaking in tongues and, at its core, a deliverance ceremony for patients. The idea of deliverance is that an evil spirit that must consequently be cast out can cause illness. Through the power of the Holy Spirit the spirits considered responsible for the mental illness are forced to manifest themselves in the patient. The spirits become discernable for the Deliverance Minister[14] through the movements and utterances in which they are embodied (cf. Meyer 1999a: Ch. 6, Csordas 2002 (1990): 64ff, Krause 2003).

In the Fellowship's way of thinking, biomedical treatment and the exorcising of demons are not mutually exclusive. Indeed its members feel that both types of treatment must be applied in order to effect a cure. According to the explanations of Dr Kanyi mental illness is multicausal in origin: lurking in the background could be, for example, a hereditary predisposition, unrecognised or wrongly treated somatic ailments (e.g., typhus that had not been completely cured, brain tumors), neuronal injuries and environmental factors (stress, marriage problems, poverty, drugs). In fact, these particular explanations correspond to international biomedical standards, as they are formulated, e.g., in the *International Classification of Diseases* (ICD-10). Yet that someone might have a genetic predisposition, is taking drugs or having marriage problems would be attributed to spiritual causes by the Fellowship. In that logic, when an evil spirit, for one reason or another, gains 'entry' into a person, then he produces, e.g., surplus dopamine that then triggers psychoses. In the words of the group's leader:

> Science can treat and only God can heal. (...) The demon who is causing the imbalance of the dopamine in your brain should be removed through healing prayer through Christ. So we believe in this Fellowship that we have to command the spirit behind your disease to go.[15]

Another relation of affinity becomes visible if one takes a closer look at how the spirits are linked to mental illness. Adapting the book *Pigs in the Parlor: A Practical Guide to Deliverance*, written by the Baptist couple Frank and Ida Mae Hammond from Texas in 1973,[16] the Fellowship conceptualises a specific demon or demon group responsible for each mental disorder. Whereas the Hammonds name the fifty three identified groups according to mental states, moods and particular characters, the Ghanaian group adds various local spirits and religious practices devoted to local gods. Another local characteristic seems to be the demonic kingdom under the sea, headed by the seductive spirit of *Mami Wata* where luxurious goods are produced, political affairs are directed and where the demons have to be sent when eventually cast out.[17] The biomedical terms used in the book of the Hammonds are taken from psychiatric vocabulary. For example, they introduce such a broad category like 'mental illness' and also a more specific single group called 'schizophrenia' (Hammond and Hammond 1973: 21).

Another central feature that appears in both the Hammonds' book and the ceremonies offered by the Fellowship, namely the demonic spiritual heritage, significantly corresponds to biomedical ideas about hereditary prepositions which could lead to mental illness. In general the tendency to identify single pathological categories and to relate them to single demonic spirits understood as transculturally valid entities, could be interpreted as the basic principle of affinity of both the biomedical treatment and the Charismatic healing.

Affinal relations between Christian healing and biomedical treatment are further created through the everyday practices of the members, most of them nurses and clinical staff. In their self-representation, each of them carries the Holy Spirit around with him or herself, praying whenever it seems necessary and thereby 'living their belief'. To them the prayers or the name Jesus are something like a 'spiritual disinfectant' against evil spirits which could jump from the patients over to the nurses and caretakers. In the words of Mary*, a nurse and member of the Fellowship:

> Before you go to the patients, you pray, because you don't know the background of the patient. We Africans, before we end up in the hospital, we might go through so many things, visit a lot of fetish shrines taking in so many concoctions. (…) The patient is already possessed. So the persons are spirited before they enter a hospital. So what will you do as a nurse? You will go and pray for that person. But you have to be very careful. You could even meet the demons that possess the patient and they will possess you. (…) So they can tempt you in the spirit to see if you are strong enough. And when you are not strong enough, you always have to ask for help of the Holy Spirit. Otherwise you are in danger.[18]

Through the elaboration of a specific discourse on development and progress and its connection to Charismatic Christianity, another affinity is articulated. In every service and prayer meeting the Holy Spirit is called to fight against obstacles which have been on the biomedical and development cooperation agenda for a long time: poverty, corruption, sickness, barrenness, suicide, the poor condition of roads and the water supply, and any shortcomings of the technical infrastructure. With prayers, the group attempts to mobilise the Holy Spirit for relief of these burdens. The Holy Spirit is seen as a spiritual force of modernisation and therefore becoming a born-again Christian opens up the mind to fully acknowledge scientific teaching, especially with regard to health. Emily*, a student nurse expresses her understanding about the connection between the wrong religious beliefs and backwardness:

> These people don't understand scientific things! The whole of Ghana is filled with African Traditional Religion. Pouring libation: they say it is for the ancestors. It has become something, the devil has made it in such a way, that it is a fashion; you don't realise that it is evil. It is a false belief, that man has occupied the mind with so many things. And no one who has the word of God has that. My people perish because they lack knowledge. If you would know about Jesus Christ you would not go and bow before that shrine. (…) So these Africans, they believe in fetish. And I take it as they don't have the knowledge of God. And their consciousness are sealed, the evil has locked their mind so much that they are ignorant towards health education.[19]

It can be concluded from Emily's statement that the right belief provides the proper attitude towards science and in the end results in a better conduct of life. Religious belief and biomedicine are in her view not a contradiction. However, biomedicine could rather be characterised by the implicit assumption that it arrives at its diagnoses independently of social, religious, cultural and political factors (Gordon 1988). In the practice of the Fellowship this assumption becomes blurred through the Christian interpretation.

Significantly for biomedical psychiatry and Christian healing is the strong impetus on a specific conduct of life which is propagated in order to gain health or to ensure the status of being born again respectively: to restrain from drugs and adultery and any sexual practice marked as deviant, to gain control over the affairs of daily life, to live self responsibly and reasonably. Using the tri-angled body model of Lock and Scheper-Hughes (1996) (see also Johannessen this volume) one could argue that the *social body* becomes the terrain where biomedical and Christian *body politics* have to be acted out in the dramatic events of deliverance to gain a new *individual body* freed from bounds that are ascribed to result from the 'unhealthy past'.

At the core of its practice, Christian Charismatic healing is directed against so-called 'traditional culture' which could be related to this construct of the 'unhealthy past'. Following this doctrine some scholars have analysed the rhetorical and ritual practice of Ghanaian Charismatic Christianity in relation to a 'conversion to modernity' especially with regard to the practice of deliverance (Gifford 1994, Meyer 1998, 1999b: Ch. 6, van Dijk 1997, 2001). Although this interpretation has been criticised (see, for example, Englund and Leach 2000, reply from Meyer 2000) it points to the important aspect, that to become a 'born again' requires 'a complete break with the past' (Meyer 1998). However, the question is, whether this past which is constructed against the here and now of salvation, could be seen as a counterpart to modernity. As I will argue in the case study below, deliverance seems to be rather an evaluation of the capacity of spirits in moral terms than a conversion to modernity.

In regard to the three dimensions of subjectivity proposed by Werbner (2002) mentioned in the beginning, the praxis of the Fellowship could be analysed as follows: The *political dimension* works through the body politics imposed on the patients. These are represented, apart from clinic routine and drug medication, in the concepts of a specific conduct of life aiming towards a governed self, dissolution from family tradition and influences, which are regarded as spiritually and psychologically unhealthy. These aspects again are closely linked to the *existential* and *moral dimensions* of the patient's situations, as will be shown in the following case example of a female patient. Her existential and social problems – how to survive socially and economically with mental sickness – have to be linked to the questions how conflicts between her family (the 'traditional past') on the one hand and the Christian doctrine (the 'healthy and modern present') on the other are expressed in her narration.

Elizabeth*: about good and about evil spirits

Elizabeth* is forty five years old and has five children born out of wedlock. The reason for her hospitalisation at the time of my research was a suicide attempt as well as aggressive behaviour and her propensity to strip naked in public. Her biomedical diagnosis is 'chronic schizophrenia', her Christian diagnosis 'possession with *Mami Wata* and other demonic spirits'. Since her first clinical treatment at age fifteen she has had several relapses into behaving *bodam*, a term used in the local language, Twi, for behaviour which violates social norms and appropriate behaviour like stripping naked publicly. Following the clinical records and the judgment of the clinical staff a strong genetic disposition for schizophrenia in her family could be assumed, because there had been other members of the family diagnosed schizophrenic as well. This assumed hereditary disposition corresponds with the Christian diagnosis and Elizabeth's subjective explanations of her illness explained below.

In the clinic she was treated with psycho pharmaceuticals and was kept calm in the female ward. Although the clinic does not offer any psychotherapy because of the lack of finance, the daily routine in the wards stabilised her: she got food three times a day and was looked after by the staff, who tried to do a kind of therapy by means of conversation. Yet apart from washing clothes, playing *oware*[20] waiting for food and medicaments, the patients have no entertainment. Therefore the healing prayer provides a bit of variety in the boring routine of the wards, especially through its elements of dancing, music and singing. Elizabeth attended the healing prayer regularly and enjoyed especially its expressive parts.

The healing prayer takes place in the entrance hall once a week in the afternoon when the Outpatient Department is closed. The nurses arrange benches along the wall and bring drums. The patients who are able to walk and who like to participate come from the wards properly dressed, the women with headscarves and in skirts, the men nicely shaved and in ironed shirts. The programme of the prayer is not fixed. It depends on the actors involved. Songs are always eligible to interrupt the flow and to give a new direction to the whole performance. Members of the Fellowship direct praying and drumming. Prayers turn most of the time into speaking in tongues by all, with raised hands, sobbing and chanting, babbling of voices. These expressive elements of praying and praises alternate during the whole event. If a member of the Fellowship who is fond of preaching is present, an interpretation of a Bible reading is given. An important element that always takes place is a special written prayer called *breaking of curses*, which is directed against spiritual heredity causing illness over the generations. The patients are lined up in a row and repeat the words. Another central feature is the deliverance. Some members of the Fellowship – the so-called Deliverance Minister – moisturise their hands with consecrated olive oil and approach every patient in the row. One minister touches the foreheads of the patients; the other two stand behind him and 'in Jesus' name' call upon the spirits who have caused the sickness to leave. All participants support the Deliverance Minister with considerable singing and drumming to invoke the power of the Holy Spirit. The belief is that the Holy Spirit should work through the hands and prayers of the Deliverance Ministers in causing the evil spirits to manifest themselves publicly. This is what happened in Elizabeth's case. She received her deliverance in a dramatic manifestation of various spirits, which could be interpreted at first sight as a moral submission to the doctrine of the Fellowship, which aims to identify the spirits in order to drive them out. One spirit, identified as a *Mami Wata* spirit coming from the sea, caused her to coil restlessly on the ground like a snake under the anointment and to dance wildly in indecent manner. Another one, who happened to be a spirit from her own family, made her strongly resist the anointed hands of the deliverance ministers and call them bad names.

We met afterwards and she explained to me what kind of spirits had manifested themselves and had caused her sickness and general misfortune. It then became clear that she acknowledged part of the doctrine, even testified to it, but at the same time told a different story. One of the spirits was *Mami Wata* who showed herself dancing titillatingly. This spirit was generally to blame for Elizabeth's unhappiness in relationships with men. *Mami Wata*, as mentioned above, is a spirit from the sea who is associated with luxurious, modern and extravagant living, prostitution and involvement with foreigners.[21] She enters spiritual marriages with human beings and thus prevents stable relationships with potential marriage partners as in the case of Elizabeth, who has never had a stable relationship, yet five children from different men.

She also talked about having inside of her the spirit of a good *abotia*.[22] This spirit was speaking impudently to the Deliverance Ministers but would be actually supporting her by saying, 'Go and do it, I will help you!' Additionally she claims that there are other bad *mmotia* and that conflict between the good and the bad spirits has caused her aggressive behaviour, leading to her hospitalisation. *Mmotia* in Twi are understood as helping spirits from the forest that represent an inversion to human beings: they walk, e.g., with feet pointed backwards. They like to be rude and to play jokes (Debrunner 1959, Field 1960). In the course of my conversation with Elizabeth it turned out, that the 'good' *abotia* (the one inside her) is holding a shrine in her family that means the spirit and the members of the family stay in a reciprocal relationship to each other which is directed by a medium (cf. Osei 1999: 27ff). When the medium or *akomfo* of the family shrine died, Elizabeth became involved in the question of his successor. The training to become a medium, an *akomfo*, consists among other things in establishing a permanent stable relationship with the respective spiritual forces (cf. Seebode 1998: 70). If these forces have not been 'socialised,' then they are experienced as disorders and difficult personal crises. Thus Elizabeth's sickness could traditionally be seen as a spiritual one which marks her out to be called the new spirit medium of the family shrine. Elizabeth resisted this call, however, in line with the Christian Charismatic discourse which assumes the *mmotia*, like all the local spirits, are demons, so that in the end their media (*akomfo*, fetish priests) are agents of Satan.

The *abotia* could be seen as representing the hereditary element of her sickness. In the biomedical sense, her father's family was assumed to be burdened by the predisposition of schizophrenia because her father's sister had the same diagnosis. In the Christian sense a family shrine represents a source of curses and evil forces that have to be fought in the above-mentioned prayer *breaking of curses*. The main goal of the Christian Charismatic deliverance as practiced by the Fellowship is to chase away all the disease-bringing spirits – in the case of Elizabeth *Mami Wata* and the *abotia* spirit – and to replace them with the one, good Holy Spirit. It essentially contrasts with the concepts of the possession priests (*akomfo*) who advocate that out of a disharmony with the spirits a reciprocal relationship with them must be forged. The disease-bringing and the healing spirits are in this case one and the same. Whereas in the Christian Charismatic concept good and evil are diametrically opposed to each other, in the *akomfo* concept these are located on a continuum. In accordance with the latter idea, a spirit, which has brought about disorder should not be chased away but pacified instead.

From an analytical perspective Elizabeth's spirits could be understood as forming aspects of her *social body* (e.g., her family) that is affected by her sickness as well. Following this view, Elizabeth's relationship to *Mami Wata* and the *mmotia* is to be interpreted in the context of her social situation. Not all the spirits in her narrative are associated with negative forces, for there is a good *abotia* spirit who is holding a shrine in her family. This can be interpreted as follows: If she accepted the *mmotia* only to be evil, this would mean a complete break with her family, which as a single mother with five children who is also stigmatised by mental illness she could not survive at all, neither socially nor economically. Her adherence to the 'good *abotia*' indicates that she regards herself as a Christian but with her self-reproaches nevertheless attached to the coping solutions offered within the family system.

This differentiates the ideology represented by the group in the clinic and the common interpretations of the Charismatic groups and churches in recent literature. The authors hardly take into account the subjective appropriations and the subjunctive aspects of conversion processes which are articulated *through* the Christian ideology and not against it. Most theories explain the growing success of the various groups and churches that have been emerging since the 1990s rather as follows: the groups claim to offer a specific blueprint for life that focuses on freeing oneself from the obligations of the extended family and on dissociating oneself from the forms of life and social practices commonly deemed 'traditional' (Marshall 1991, Gifford 1994, Meyer 1995, 1998, 1999a, van Dijk 2001). However, Elizabeth's case tells a different story without rejecting the Christian message. She recounts that the good *abotia* did not leave her, but stays with her as a good companion:

> I suppose within my heart it is a good one. (...) They drive him away. So he came outside from me, beside me. (...) He becomes a friend of mine! I don't see him, but he will accompany me. But I will not allow him to come back into my heart, only Jesus is in my heart.

This shows that the spirit of the one *abotia*, the spiritual head of her family, remains a positive force in regard to her future life. She declares him to be a companion. From what I found out about the circumstances of her life, it is clear that her family supports her and, for instance, helps to care for her children. This can nowadays no longer be taken for granted in Ghana, where the fulfillment of social obligations within a family has become increasingly rare as here, too, more and more areas of society have become exposed to the exploitative logic of capitalism and of global competition. Thus individual family members who may have managed to accumulate a bit of wealth are becoming ever more frequently saddled with the burden of having to share it with increasing numbers of ever poorer relatives. Elizabeth's story represents the absolute prototype of a great burden, especially when we recall that her disorder began so early in life, meaning that she has repeatedly been seriously ill and dependent on family support. Therefore her agency is articulated through and not against the moral order of the family.

In contrast to the *abotia*, the *Mami Wata* spirit is to be found outside of what is defined as the familial social sphere and is classified as belonging to the 'foreigners who come over the sea' – (Twi for Europeans: *aborofo*) i.e., to the Europeans (Drewal 1988: 161). The wealth from her realm on the sea bed that she promises to her followers is individually acquired wealth in contrast to inherited property wealth. As Henry Drewal points out, in promising to her disciples a carefree luxurious life unencumbered by social obligations, *Mami Wata* has opened up new ranges of activities in the postcolonial capitalistic society, an appropriation of Western consumer goods and life styles (Drewal 1988: 161). Yet as Birgit Meyer has described in her works (1999a: 210; 1999b), these very things have also been striven for by the Charismatic Christians, but their relationship towards the so-called modern lifestyle on the whole has nevertheless remained highly ambivalent. For the Charismatic Christians the negative aspect of modern life is virtually personified in *Mami Wata*, as it is vividly expressed in the growingly popular Christian media products, like video films or booklets. *Mami Wata* riches are portrayed as the bait that leads straightaway into the clutches of Evil.

Since social climbing and luxury goods are out of the question for Elizabeth because of her situation, it is no problem for her to have *Mami Wata* (but not the *abotia*) chased back into the sea. Hence she agrees, in the case of *Mami Wata*, with the spirit's condemnation as practiced by the Charismatic Christians but keeps the friendly *abotia* beside her. Thus she interprets aspects of her illness which have a different meaning in the biomedical discourse (the illusion of hearing a voice), and the Christian Charismatic (an evil spirit, tied to her through the history of her family and therefore to be cast out) in a subjunctive mode: her aim is to find out how to go on in the future and how to deal with her chronic sickness.

Conclusion

At one and the same time Elizabeth consents to and is confused by the *body politics* imposed on her by the Christian Charismatic healing and the biomedical treatment. To express her concerns she uses both of the complementary discourses offered. On the one hand, she embraces both practices. This could be seen in her subjugation to the *body politics* in the form of participating in the daily routine of the ward, accepting its regulating effects and taking willingly the prescribed drugs. In addition, she insists on the existence of her spirits and interprets them in the religious realm offered by the Fellowship. On the other hand, in both instances she only partly adapts to the system. She is absorbing and transforming it at the same time. She takes drugs, undergoes deliverances but also keeps the spirit who can serve as a supporting companion next to her. She articulates that 'only Jesus' is 'in her heart', which could be seen as adequate to the doctrine propagated by the Fellowship but, at the same time also stays in good relation with the family spirit, the *abotia*. Following the biomedical discourse it must be acknowledged that there are no spirits speaking to her, but that these voices are illusions. Furthermore, in biomedical thinking, the assumption of the heard voices of spirits like the *abotia* could become 'rhetorical core devices' (Kleinman 1995: 22) and could lead in the end to the diagnosis of a psychotic state. The principal distinction between a system of illusions and a religious belief system consist of the fact that illusions are idiosyncratic experiences and visions are acknowledged in a shared meaning system of a religious group. It could be assumed that the Christian Fellowship in its syncretistic practice provides a frame within which patients could articulate in a subjunctive mood their situated concerns, even if they do it through spirits (Krause 2003).

The various contested spirits are thematic representations of conflicts that in no way belong to the past or contradict biomedical treatment, but are acute in the here and now of society (Luig 1999). The story of Elizabeth can be understood concerning the dimensions of subjectivity mentioned above by Werbner. The message Elizabeth took out of the Charismatic ideology was *moral* (valuating good and evil spirits) and not so much a question of conversion to modernity. Nevertheless, the self-representation of the Charismatic groups could (mis)lead to the latter interpretation. Most significant in this regard seems to be the strong neo-liberal message contained in the sermons and pamphlets of the Charismatic movement. This can be related to the *political* dimension of her appropriation as well as the body politics that goes along with it. Elizabeth undergoes the specific interactive situation of deliverance and undertakes the decision to keep the one *abotia* spirit and not to chase him away. As the story of Elizabeth shows, her choice to subject herself to certain spirits and body politics emerges from the necessity to undertake an *existential* valuation (the third dimension of subjectivity that Werbner mentions) of the possibilities: to undergo isolation from her family or to undertake interaction with humans and spirits.

In the practice of the Fellowship we find no contradiction of religion and medicine but rather a conflicted relationship of contested spirits between different religious healing methods and a complementary relation between drugs and anointment. It could be assumed that, because of the variety of affinal relations between Charismatic Christianity and biomedical psychiatry, and because of the ongoing success of this religious movement, this combination will be of some significance for a possible restructuring of the pluralistic medical scene, not only in Ghana, but in other African countries as well.

Within the competitive scene of alternative healing methods the Christian discourse is demonising the other religious practices. This is true according to the message spread by the Fellowship and popular Christian discourse. However, the narratives of patients like Elizabeth contradict these ideological incompatibilities. In the material presented we find an intricate tying together of the various interpretations of the illness and treatment possibilities utilised by the actors involved. To express it differently: as the case example shows, even if someone takes pills, spirits can still be seen as part of a meaningful process of construing sickness and healing.

Notes

1. In Medical Anthropology the reference to 'experience' became very prominent. In my opinion this does not provide a real solution because it contains problematic epistemological pre-assumption: that we could get access to the real thing – experience – and that we could get to know about this experience independently of the relations between subject and the processes of subjugation itself. The recent revival of narrative analysis in Medical Anthropology draws heavily on the notion of experience (cf. Mattingly and Garro 2000, Skultans 2000, for a critical comment Atkinson 1997). In contrast, the work of Allan Young shows how narrated experiences are already devoted to as well as used and shaped by discourses (Young 1993, 1995). I share Young's scepticism, especially concerning medical settings. However, as long we are carrying out qualitative research which is concerned with actors who 'undergo and undertake' we need to struggle with the problem. I regard the project of this volume as a contribution to this challenge.

2. I am grateful to my colleagues Viktoria Bergschmidt, Iris Meilicke and Katharina Schramm for critical and helpful discussions and to the editors of this volume for their comments. My thanks are also extended to Johanna Hoornweg for polishing my English.

3. Research was carried out from June 1998 to the end of February 1999 and was funded by a scholarship from the Friedrich-Ebert Stiftung.

4. Drawing on her longstanding research on misfortune, affliction (cf. 1997) and specifically on AIDS, Whyte is concerned with how people come to terms with extreme uncertainties. 'Subjunctivity is not a characteristic of the times. It is about the specific uncertainty that particular actors experience as they try something that matters to them – as they undertake to deal with a problem. That is to say, it is a mood of the verb, it is about action, and especially interaction' (Whyte 2002: 175). Cf. Good 1994: 153ff who used the term 'subjunctive mood' first but in a slightly different way.

5. Broadly referring to the concept of appropriation (in German *Aneignung*) in Marxist theory, the term is understood here as creative acts and practices which empower persons. In the process of appropriation the appropriated and the person herself become changed.

6. Els van Dongen (2002) invented this term for her analyses of narrations of psychotic patients.

7. Several projects aiming to initiate cooperation at the primary healthcare level were carried out in Ghana and are still on the agenda. For an overview and a re-evaluation see Ventevogel 1996.

8. In the last years the Ministry of Health started to attach so-called psychiatric units to the regional hospitals to improve the basic psychiatric care.

9. Cf. Twumasi 1975, 1979; Osei 1999. For an overview of the religious history of Ghana see Assimeng 1986, 1995; Sackey 2001 for the different Christian churches.
10. Concerning the demonising discourse of the new Christian groups see Meyer (1998, 1999a).
11. There has been a boom of literature on Charismatic Christianity in the last years. For an in depth' overview on African Christianity in general, see Meyer 2004; on Ghana, Meyer 1995, 1996, 1998, 1999a, 1999b, Gifford 1994 and van Dijk 1997, 2001; on Latin America and Africa, the contributions in the volume edited by Corton and Marshall-Fratani 2001; with regard to aspects of globalisation and transnational Christian networks, see Coleman 2002.
12. Corinthians 12: 7–11, 14: 1–9; Luke 9: 1, 6; Matthew 10: 1–10; Mark 6: 7–13; John 14: 15, 25f.
13. All names with * are changed, but the * will only appear the first time the name is mentioned. His spiritual approach to mental illness was regarded as 'hypnotism' by the principal psychiatrist of the Ministry of Health. Other colleagues sometimes referred patients to him who, in example, are convinced they are victims of witchcraft.
14. Deliverance Ministers are experts of the groups who are qualified through the gifts of the Holy Spirit. Most of them are men, because they are assumed to be stronger than women in resisting the evil spirits.
15. Dr Kanyi teaching in English at the Healing and Fasting Prayer session of 1 August 1998.
16. Translated into Spanish and printed in thirty six editions. See for the transnational circulation Bastian 2002: ref. 5. Numerous Christian homepages recommend it.
17. Meyer 1995, 1996, 1999b, 2002 and Bastian 1998, 2002 have written about Mami Wata and the riches from the sea, especially about how this imagery is used in popular culture like video films and booklets. Gifford (2001) criticises the underestimation of the strong influence of North American ideologies on the spread of African Charismatic Christians. However, the demonic kingdom under the sea provides an example of the transnational circulation of imageries from Africa to the United States, too. As an 'African thread' it becomes acknowledged especially through the circulation of Nigerian tracts like Eni 1987 and Uzorma 1994 in recent North American publications; see http://www.demonbuster.com/znigerian.html (1 April 2003).
18. Interview Mary in English, 6 August 1998.
19. Interview Emily in English 2 August 1998. Especially in such a quotation it becomes evident, how contested the notion of 'African' and 'tradition' becomes in the Charismatic discourse. 'These Africans' seem not to include 'me, the Christian'. With Fanon (2000) in mind, the self-fulfilment becomes self-neglecting in the postcolonial situation. Therefore Ghanaian intellectuals heavily criticise this new religious movement.
20. Popular African board game.
21. Cf. Kramer 1987, Drewal 1988. See Wendl 1991: chapter 3 and 4, O'Brien Wicker 2000: 209ff for Ewe priests in Ghana. In relation to Charismatic Christianity in Ghana cf. Meyer 1999a, Ch. 7, and her recent work on Mami Wata in video films (Meyer 2002).
22. Twi: 'short people', sometimes also translated as 'dwarf'; plural form *mmotia*.

References

Atkinson, P. 1997: 'Narrative Turn or Blind Alley?' *Qualitative Health Research* 7(3): 325–44.

Assimeng, M. 1986. *Saints and Social Structures*. Accra: Accra-Tema.

Assimeng, M. 1995. 'Salvation, Social Crisis and the Human Condition'. Inaugural Lecture delivered at the University of Ghana on 27 July 1989. Accra.

Bastian, M. 1998. 'Mami Wata, Mr. White, and the Sirens Off Bar Beach: Spirits and Dangerous Consumption in the Nigerian Popular Press', in H. Schmidt and A. Wirtz (eds) *Afrika und das Andere. Alterität und Innovation*. Münster: LIT Verlag, 21–31.

——2002. 'Take the Battle to the Enemies' Camp: Militarizing the Spirit in Nigerian Pentecostal Christianity'. Paper presented at the panel: 'Spiritual Warfare: Religion and Conflict in Africa', AAA Annual Meeting, Nov. 2002, New Orleans.

Butler, J. 1993. *Bodies That Matter*. New York, London: Routledge.

Coleman, S. 2002. 'The Faith Movement: a Global Religious Culture?' *Culture and Religion. An Interdisciplinary Journal* 3(1): 3–19.

Corton, A. and R. Marshall-Fratani (eds) 2001. *Between Babel and Pentecost. Transnational Pentecostalism in Africa and Latin America*. Bloomington, Indianapolis: Indiana University Press.

Csordas, T.J. 2002. *Body/Meaning/Healing*. New York: Palgrave.

Debrunner, H.W. 1959. *Witchcraft in Ghana. A Study on the Belief in Destructive Witches and its Effect on the Akan Tribes*. Kumasi: Presbyterian Book Depot.

Drewal, H.J. 1988. 'Performing the Other. Mami Wata Worship in Africa', *The Drama Review* 32(2): 160–185.

Englund, H. and J. Leach. 2000. 'Ethnography and the Meta-narratives of Modernity', *Current Anthropology* 41(2): 225–239.

Eni, E. 1987. *Delivered from the Power of Darkness*. Ibadan, Nigeria: Scripture Union.

Fanon, F. 2000 (1952). *Black Skin White Masks*. London: Pluto.

Field, M.J. 1960. *Search for Security. An Ethnopsychiatric Study of Rural Ghana*. London: Faber and Faber.

Fink, H.E. 1987. *Religion, Disease and Healing in Ghana*. München: Trickster Wissenschaft.

Foucault, M. 1972 (1961). *Histoire de la folie à l'age classique*. Paris: Gallimard.

Gifford, P. 1994. Ghana's Charismatic Churches, *Journal of Religion in Africa*, 24(3): 241–265.

——2001: 'The Complex Provenance of Some Elements of African Pentecostalism', in A. Corten and R. Marshall-Fratani (eds) *Between Babel and Pentecost. Transnational Pentecostalism in Africa and Latin America*. Bloomington, Indianapolis, Indiana University Press, 62–79.

Gordon, D. 1988. 'Tenacious Assumptions in Western Medicine', in M. Lock and D. Gordon (eds) *Biomedicine Examined*. Dordrecht: Kluwer, 19–56.

Good, B. 1994. *Medicine, Rationality and Experience. An Anthropological Perspective*. Cambridge: Cambridge University Press.

Hammond, F. and I. Hammond. 1973. *Pigs in the Parlor. A Practical Guide to Deliverance*. Kirkwood: Impact Books.

Kleinman, A. 1995. *Writing at the Margin. Discourse between Anthropology and Medicine*. Berkeley, Los Angeles, London: University of California Press.

Kramer, F. 1987. *Der rote Fes. Über Besessenheit und Kunst in Afrika*. Frankfurt/Main: Athenäum.

Krause, K. 2003. 'Der Heilige Geist und die Geister. Christliche Heilbehandlungen in einem psychiatrischen Krankenhaus in Süd-Ghana.' Unpublished MA Thesis, Free University Berlin, Department for Social Anthropology.

Lambek, M. 2002. 'Nuriaty, the Saint and the Sultan. Virtuous Subjects and Subjective Virtuoso of the Postmodern Colony', in R. Werbner (ed.) *Postcolonial Subjectivities in Africa*. London and New York: Zed Books, 25–43.

Lock, M. and N. Scheper-Hughes. 1996. 'A Critical-interpretative Approach in Medical Anthropology: Rituals and Routines of Discipline and Dissent', in C.F.

Sargent and T.M. Johnson (eds) *Medical Anthropology. Contemporary Theory and Method*. Westport and London: Praeger, 41–70.

Luig, U. 1999. 'Constructing Local Worlds. Spirit Possession in the Gwembe Valley. Zambia', in H. Behrend and U. Luig (eds) *Spirit Possession, Modernity and Power in Africa*. London: James Currey Publishers, 124–141.

Marshall, R. 1991. 'Power in the Name of Jesus', *Review of African Political Economy* 52: 21–37.

Mattingly, C. and L.C. Garro (eds) 2000. *Narrative and the Cultural Construction of Illness and Healing*. Berkeley: University of California Press.

Meyer, B. 1995. 'Delivered from the Powers of Darkness. Confessions about Satanic Riches in Christian Ghana', *Africa* 65(2): 236–255.

——1996. 'Modernity and Enchantement: the Image of the Devil in Popular African Christianity', in P. van der Veer (ed.) *Conversion to Modernities: the Globalization of Christianity*. London and New York: Routledge.

——1998. 'Make a Complete Break with the Past: Memory and Postcolonial Modernity in Ghanaian Pentecostalist Discourse', *Journal of Religion in Africa* 28(3): 316–349.

——1999a. *Translating the Devil. Religion and Modernity Among the Ewe in Ghana*. Edinburg: Edinburg University Press. Africa World Press Inc.

——1999b. 'Commodities and the Power of Prayer: Pentecostalists Attitudes towards Consumption in Contemporary Ghana', in B. Meyer and P. Geschiere (eds) *Globalization and Identity: Dialectics of Flow and Closure*. Oxford: Blackwell, 151–76.

——2000. 'Comment on Englund and Leach: "Ethnography and the Meta-Narratives of Modernity"', *Current Anthropology* 41(2): 241–242.

——2002. 'Pentecostalism, Prosperity and Popular Cinema in Ghana', *Culture and Religion*, 3 (1): 67–87.

——2004. 'Christianity in Africa: From African Independent to Pentecostal-Charismatic Churches', *Annual Review of Anthropology*, 33: 447–474.

Mullings, L. 1984. *Therapy, Ideology and Social Change. Mental Healing in Urban Ghana*. Berkeley, Los Angeles, London: University of California Press.

O'Brien Wicker, K. 2000. 'Mami Water in African Religion and Spirituality', in J.K. Olupona (ed.) *African Spirituality. Forms, Meanings and Expressions*. New York: Crossroad, 198–222.

Osei, A.O. 1999. 'Prevalence of Psychiatric Morbidity among Patients Attending three Traditional Healing Centres in the Ashanati Region of Ghana.' Dissertation, West African College of Physicians, Faculty of Psychiatry, University of Science and Technology, Kumasi.

Osei, Y. 1997. 'Psychiatrische Einrichtungen in einem Entwicklungsland – das Beispiel Ghana', in K. Hoffman and W. Machleidt (eds) *Psychiatrie im Kulturvergleich*. Berlin: Verlag für Wissenschaft und Bildung, 131–137.

Rose, N. 1992a. 'Governing the Enterprising Self', in P. Heelas and P. Morris (eds) *The Values of the Enterprise Culture. The Moral Debate*. London and New York: Routledge, 141–164.

——1992b. 'Of Madness itself. Histoire de la folie and the object of psychiatric history', in A. Still and I. Velody (eds) *Rewriting the History of Madness. Studies in Foucaults Histoire de la folie*. London, New York: Routledge, 142–149.

Sackey, B. 2001. 'Charismatics, Independents, and Missions: Church Proliferation in Ghana', *Culture and Religion* 2(1): 41–59.

Seebode, J. 1998. '"*Aduro kum aduro*" - *Ritual, Macht und Besessenheit in Asante (Südghana')*. Hamburg: Lit Verlag.

Skultans, V. 2000. 'Narrative Illness and the Body', *Anthropology & Medicine* 7(1): 5–12.

Twumasi, P.A. 1975. *Medical Systems in Ghana. A Study in Medical Sociology.* Accra: Accra-Tema.

———1979: A Social History of the Ghanaian Pluralistic Medical System, *Social Science & Medicine* 13b: 349–56.

Uzorma, I.N. 1994. *Occult Grand Master Now in Christ.* Uzorma Warefare Treatise book One. Lagos, Nigeria: Franco-Bon Publishing Ministry.

van Dijk, R. 1997. 'From Camp to Encompassment: Discourses of Transsubjectivity in the Ghanaian Pentecostal Diaspora', *Journal of Religion in Africa* 27(2): 135–169.

———2001 'Contesting Silence: the Ban on Drumming and the Musical Politics of Pentecostalism in Ghana', *Ghana Studies* 4: 31–64.

van Dongen, E. 2002. *Walking Stories. An Oddnography of Mad People's Work With Culture.* Amsterdam: Rozenberg.

Ventevogel, P. 1996. *Whiteman's Things. Training and Detraining Healers in Ghana.* Amsterdam: Het Spinhuis.

Wendl, T. 1991. *Mami Wata oder ein Kult zwischen den Kulturen.* Münster: Lit Verlag.

Werbner, R. 2002. 'Introduction: Postcolonial Subjectivities: The Personal, the Political and the Moral', in R. Werbner (ed.) *Postcolonial Subjectivities in Africa.* London and New York: Zed Books, 1–21.

Whyte, S.R. 1989. 'Anthropological Approaches to African Misfortune: From Religion to Medicine', in A. Jacobsen-Widding and D. Westerlund (eds) *Culture, Experience and Pluralism: Essays on African Ideas of Illness and Healing.* Uppsala: Uppsala University, 289–301.

———1997. *Questioning Misfortune. The Pragmatics of Uncertainty in Eastern Uganda.* Cambridge: Cambridge University Press.

———2002. 'Subjectivity and Subjunctivity. Hoping for Health in Eastern Uganda', in Werbner, R. (ed.) *Postcolonial Subjectivities in Africa,* London and New York: Zed Books, 171–190.

Wolf, A. and M. Stürzer (eds) 1996. *Die gesellschaftliche Konstruktion von Befindlichkeit. Ein Sammelband zur Medizinethnologie.* Berlin: Verlag für Wissenschaft und Bildung.

Young, A. 1993. 'A Description of How Ideology Shapes Knowledge of a Mental Disorder (Posttraumatic Stress Disorder)', in S. Lindenbaum and M. Lock (eds) *Knowledge, Power, and Practice. The Anthropology of Medicine and Everyday Life,* Berkeley, Los Angeles. London: University of California Press, 108–144.

———1995. *The Harmony of Illusions. Inventing Post-Traumatic Stress Disorder.* Princeton: Princeton University Press.

5

German Medical Doctors' Motives for Practising Homoeopathy, Acupuncture or Ayurveda

Robert Frank and Gunnar Stollberg

Perhaps the most obvious questions that arise when surprising social developments occur are: 'Who are these people? And why are they doing it?' As regards the (re-) emergence of heterodox medicine in Europe and North America during the last two decades, numerous studies were conducted to answer these two questions. Most of these studies were concerned with the patients' perspectives: Patients often turn to heterodox medicine if they suffer from non-life-threatening chronic diseases for which biomedical treatment has produced unwanted side-effects rather than an effective cure. Therefore, the promise of gentle healing in heterodox medicine is appealing (Furnham and Smith 1988, Sharma 1990). Another type of heterodox patient has ideas on health that more closely correspond with heterodox treatment than with biomedicine (Stollberg 2002). It has been argued that heterodox patients were alienated from biomedical forms of the physician-patient relationship (Fairclough 1992). Empirical evidence of harmonious interactions in heterodox medicine is, however, ambiguous (Frank 2002a). Much less is known about the motives of those *practising* heterodox medicine (Cant and Sharma 1999). Sharma (1992) presented a wide range of motivational factors for non-medical practitioners, partly of a practical nature (e.g., possibility of flexible part-time work). Most of her interviewees practised another – not necessarily medical – profession before taking up heterodox medicine (Sharma 1992). We can assume that motives and career patterns are different for medical doctors practising heterodox medicine, as their professional biographies involve at least a decade of biomedical training.

Lynöe and Svensson (1992) found that physicians were disappointed with biomedicine's limited efficacy and the side-effects of biomedical drugs, and this was a major reason why medical doctors turned to heterodox medicine. Goldstein (1985) examines personal characteristics and the motives of members of the American Holistic Medical Association (AHMA). These Californian physicians reported – besides disappointment with biomedicine – various personal reasons for their change in career. Spiritual leanings, positive experiences with heterodox medicine during serious diseases or personal crises (e.g., divorce, psychotherapy) laid the foundation for their interest in heterodox medicine. One might speculate whether these results are specific to the Californian context (which is said to be more open to New Age ideas) or to the physicians' organisational body (AHMA). Goldstein et al. (1988) compare heterodox physicians to general practitioners (GP). While spiritual and religious leanings represent important differences between the two groups, the findings on personal crises and personal experiences with heterodox medicine were not confirmed. It might be worth noting that heterodox physicians earn significantly less than their biomedical colleagues (Goldstein et al. 1988). Goldstein's studies offer rich data on the characteristics of heterodox medical doctors. However, all kinds of heterodox medicine have been pooled together in these studies. Therefore, differences *within* the heterodox medical profession are invisible, and the heterogeneity of heterodox medicine is ignored. Given the wide range of heterodox modes of medicine, it would be rather surprising if one homogenous set of motives emerged.

Heterodox medical doctors deviate from a relatively secure career path and do not shy away from the economic risks that accompany heterodox medical practice (Goldstein et al. 1988). They have been described as heretics who are relentlessly persecuted and disciplined by the medical mainstream (Wolpe 1990, Dew 1997).

Apart from these empirical studies, the motives of heterodox medical doctors were studied within the framework of professionalisation theory. By analysing the strategies of the respective organisational bodies, Saks (1994) argues that the medical profession's interest in acupuncture mainly serves to fend off the 'alternative challenge' (Saks 1992). While medical doctors start practising acupuncture, non-medical acupuncturists continue to be attacked and excluded. Therefore, Saks (1995) concludes that the medical profession's increasing openness to heterodox medicine is far from being altruistic, but rather in the profession's self-interest.

In the following study, we try to compare the motives of German medical doctors in three heterodox settings: homoeopathy, acupuncture, Ayurveda. This procedure allows us to study whether there is any correlation between the different types of heterodox medicine and the motives of the respective physicians who practise them. With these considerations in mind, we try to answer our initial question: 'Who are these people? And why are they doing it?'

Methods

As there are only a few studies on the motives of heterodox physicians, the application of a qualitative, explorative research approach seemed most appropriate for this study. By conducting semi-structured interviews and posing open-ended questions that were handled flexibly, it was possible to achieve a certain degree of comparability, which was nevertheless open to any unexpected categories. There were slight variations in the sampling procedures for the three groups of physicians: Forty-two of the 105 'homoeopathic physicians' in the Yellow Pages of Berlin (1999) were randomly selected, written to once and asked to participate in this study. This led to twenty interviews, which were conducted between July and September 1999.

Acupuncturists and Ayurvedic physicians were contacted by telephone. This resulted in a participation rate of 100 percent in both groups. Medical acupuncturists were selected randomly from two different sources: The Yellow Pages Berlin and the register kept by the largest organisational body of medical acupuncturists in Germany (DÄGfA). While interviews with medical homoeopaths and acupuncturists were exclusively conducted in Berlin, a different procedure was required for Ayurveda, as there is only a small number of Ayurvedic physicians in Germany. The participants were selected from an address list on the Maharishi Ayurveda[1] website[2], while other interviewees were tracked down from all across Germany. This sampling procedure led to fourteen interviews with medical acupuncturists, and fifteen with Ayurvedic physicians.

The interviews were all conducted by Robert Frank and took place at the physicians' practices and lasted between thirty-five and eighty-five minutes. The majority of the participants were GPs, which was consistent with the generally high acceptance of heterodox medicine among this group (Tovey 1997). However, the sample also included consultants like urologists, radiologists, paediatricians and – particularly among acupuncturists – surgeons. The interviews were audio-tape recorded and transcribed. Assisted by software for qualitative data analysis, both authors independently identified key concepts. Each sequence of the interviews was coded and a system of categories was developed for the whole material along the lines of qualitative content analysis according to Mayring (1988). Further interpretation included cross-case analysis as well as individual analysis.

Germany is said to be particularly open to heterodox medicine (Cant and Sharma 1999). German public health insurance companies[3] provide some reimbursement for acupuncture and homoeopathy, while patients pay for Ayurvedic treatment privately (Frank and Stollberg 2002). Acupuncture appears to be the most accepted form of heterodox medicine in contemporary Germany. The number of members of the largest professional organisation (DÄGfA) is as great as the number of naturopathic and homoeopathic physicians combined. Homoeopathy – having been developed by the German physician S. Hahnemann (1755–1843) – has been a relatively

Table 5.1 *Membership of heterodox medical organisations in Germany 2002/2003*

Physicians in Germany (total numbers)	approx. 298,000
In their own practices/offices	approx. 122,000
Society of Physicians for Acupuncture (DÄGfA)	approx. 29,400
Central Council of Homoeopathic Physicians	approx. 4,000
Central Council of Naturopathic Physicians	approx. 11,000
Ayurvedic Physicians	approx. 140

prominent mode of treatment in Germany over the last two hundred years. The standing of Ayurveda in the German health care system is – despite its current presence in the mass media – marginal. Some one hundred physicians use Ayurveda in their practice (cf. table 5.1).

In the following, we present the reasons our participants reported for their decision to turn to heterodox medicine. A common feature in all three groups was that only a few physicians chose to take up heterodox medicine before or during their studies. The usual pattern was to opt for heterodox medicine after they had entered the professional world of biomedicine.

Medical homoeopaths

Unease with biomedicine – limited efficacy

For medical homoeopaths, the most frequently reported reason for switching to heterodox medicine was their relationship with biomedicine. These physicians were particularly disillusioned by biomedicine's therapeutic options: For them, biomedical drugs are – especially in chronic cases – rarely able to cure the patients. Biomedical therapy might be able to alleviate the patients' symptoms for a limited period of time, but a relapse is inevitable:

> I was so unhappy with what I experienced while I was working in hospital. Particularly in internal medicine! It was so sad and without any success. With chronic patients it was the worst: They came every four to six weeks, we got them back on their feet again to a certain extent with our treatment, but after a while it was the same as before. (Hom[4] 10)

> There are few occasions in biomedicine where you actually *heal*. You narcotise, you conceal, you suppress, kill bacteria for a while, but you never really enhance the health of the patient. If the blood pressure is high, it will be brought down, if it is low it will be increased. They always work according to the principle of contraries.[5] Because of this principle, the body always has to struggle against suppression. (Hom 11)

> Soon after I opened up my practice, I realised that I could only adequately treat 30 per cent of my patients by biomedical means. So, if I see ten patients within two hours, I have helped three of them. And I had to look for something for the remaining seven. (Hom 13)

From the homoeopaths' perspective, patients pay a high price for this limited therapeutic success. They regarded the side-effects of biomedical drugs as a major problem with biomedical treatment, and this led to their interest in homoeopathy:

> In hospital, the treatment could be worse than the disease. In intensive care you nearly kill people sometimes. And this was something I did not want to be part of anymore. (Hom 12)

> If you prescribe an antibiotic, I have to admit it does do its job in the short term. But patients often feel so lethargic afterwards. The infection has gone, but their vitality has suffered. (Hom 5)

These two aspects of biomedicine – the limited curative potential and the side-effects of the drugs – were evident in nearly all of the interviews with medical homoeopaths. The resultant frustration affected their job satisfaction and even led to ethical problems for some of them:

> I got to the point where I said: 'This is it. I don't want to be responsible for biomedicine anymore!' (Hom 9)

In these accounts, we have to deal with the methodological problem inherent in collecting retrospective data. The recollection of past events appears to be shaped by the participants' present perspectives (Sudman et al. 1996). Homoeopathic terminology are used to describe their experiences of how biomedicine 'suppresses' symptoms. However, while the physicians were still practising biomedicine, they were not familiar with this terminology. We might assume that their unease with biomedicine was less defined. The general impression that biomedicine's efficacy was limited, that 'the patients keep coming back' (Hom 3), might have been dominant.

Positive experience with homoeopathy

The majority of medical homoeopaths in this study underwent homoeopathic treatment themselves. For eight of them, this took place after their homoeopathic training and served to dispel remaining doubts and to confirm the efficacy of homoeopathy. Therefore, their homoeopathic experiences should not be treated as motivating factors. However, for another five of the twenty homoeopaths, the successful treatment of chronic diseases (eczema, multiple allergies) turned their general unease with biomedical practice into a specific interest in homoeopathy:

I have had eczema since I was two years old. I started homoeopathic treatment in 1989 and it was effective. This of course reinforced my curiosity about homoeopathy and I never consulted a biomedical doctor again. (Hom 6).

Two of the medical homoeopaths received homoeopathic treatment in their childhood. After becoming chronically ill as an adult, they tried out homoeopathy once more:

I went to a homoeopath when I was a boy, because biomedicine was no help to me. It was a very pleasant experience and I remembered it when I got sick many years later. The physician I went to was also teaching homoeopathy and I started the course right away. (Hom 17)

Four of the twenty participants in this study were attracted to homoeopathy after witnessing how their own patients were cured by homoeopathy while they themselves were still practising biomedicine. They described spectacular instances of healing as being integral to their conversion:

One of my patients had a chronic, recurring inflammation of the salivary gland. Nobody knew what he had. And he was cured by some of those little homoeopathic pills. I was intrigued. (Hom 14)

There was this child, very sick, and I didn't know what to do, because she developed terrible side-effects no matter what drug I tried. I gave up and told the parents: 'Try something different.' They took her to a homoeopath. Three years later, I ran into her: She received her homoeopathic remedy, was much stronger and completely healthy. Then I said to myself: 'I have to look into that.' But I still couldn't see how it could possibly work. (Hom 9)

Spirituality

One of the twenty homoeopaths in our study reported that spiritual leanings were a major reason for his interest in homoeopathy. Like his colleagues, he criticised biomedicine, but his disillusionment was less extreme as he had never expected a lot from biomedicine:

The main reason was that I have been very interested in religious and spiritual aspects of life since I was around twenty. This led me to alternative medicine, where I was looking for religion in the broadest sense. (Hom 3)

It is interesting that this physician was the only homoeopath who thought about practising heterodox medicine *before* studying medicine. He was wondering whether to become a *Heilpraktiker*[6] or a medical doctor.

The reasons that lead medical homoeopaths to practise homoeopathy appear to be firmly embedded in their professional and personal experiences: negative experiences with biomedicine, positive experiences with homoeopathy. While a certain amount of disillusionment with biomedicine was to be expected, there were only a few ideological or cultural aspects, such as a generally holistic worldview, which led to the practice of homoeopathy. It is also remarkable that all except one participant in this study did not feel alienated from biomedicine until they actually took up biomedical positions. We will see how these patterns compare to the reasons why physicians practise Asian forms of medicine like acupuncture or Ayurveda. It is these to which we now turn.

Ayurvedic physicians

Indophilia

Ayurveda is still barely recognised within the German health care system. Only around one hundred medical doctors use Ayurveda in their practice. A distinctive aspect of their motivation to do so is their personal relationship with Indian culture. Six of the fifteen Ayurvedic medical doctors interviewed in this study reported that they were drawn to Indian culture first and then became aware of Ayurveda. The attraction to Indian culture paved the way for their Ayurvedic practice:

> When did I start becoming interested in Ayurveda? Hard to say. I would prefer to say 'interested in Indian culture.' I first travelled to India in 1979 when I was twenty-one, and I was completely overwhelmed. Five years later, I went back in order to digest everything that had happened during my first trip. I was instantly fascinated by India. (Ayu[7] 5)

> I always felt close to India as my grandmother had so many paintings of India hanging on the wall. Her brother-in-law had been to Indonesia with the Dutch and was deported to the Himalayas. There he met Heinrich Harrer,[8] worked with him and prepared his escape to the Dalai Lama's place of exile. And he painted all these pictures and told so many stories. I always knew that this was where I wanted to go. So the interest in India preceded the interest in Ayurveda. (Ayu 9)

> When I was working in hospital, I also studied mythology at university. I used to do yoga – in as early as 1971 – and I knew someone who wanted to become an Indian monk, for whatever reason. The early 1970s were such a romantic period, you know. And he owned the compendia by Caraka and Susruta[9] and gave them to me. That's how it all started. (Ayu 12)

We can see how these physicians perceive Ayurveda to be intimately associated with Indian culture and philosophy. This motivational pattern corresponds with their style of medical practice. These physicians try to adopt a rather purist approach to Ayurveda, attempting to combine it as little as possible with biomedicine or other forms of heterodox medicine (Frank 2004). This correlation of practice styles and motivational patterns does not apply to medical homoeopaths. While medical homoeopaths engage in varying types of homoeopathic practice[10] (Frank 2002b), their reasons for doing so are rather homogenous.

As there are no standardised courses in Ayurveda in Germany, the physicians themselves are responsible for deciding how to acquire Ayurvedic knowledge. Most of the physicians who turned to Ayurveda because they felt an affinity for Indian culture and philosophy studied Ayurvedic writings on their own, while three of them combined this approach with extended periods of practice in Ayurvedic hospitals in India. One of them even obtained a Bachelor of Ayurvedic Medicine and Surgery (BAMS) in India after her graduation from medicine.

Existing practice of heterodox medicine

Unlike homoeopathy, where different experiences reinforced each other, we find different motives among Ayurvedic physicians. The participants in our study reported *either* their affinity with Indian culture *or* an existing attraction to heterodox medicine. Nine of the fifteen physicians had already practised Western or Asian forms of heterodox treatment before becoming aware of Ayurveda. Therefore, turning to Ayurveda did not open up a completely new career path for them as it did for 'indophile' Ayurvedic physicians or medical homoeopaths. Instead, it extended the range of heterodox methods that they offered to their patients:

> I believe you have to be born to practise in this way, and this includes having a passion for nature and naturopathy. You see, I grew up in the countryside. My mother used to treat me with herbs and later I went to extra courses in homoeopathy and acupuncture while I was studying medicine. (Ayu 13)

> The foundations were already laid by acupuncture and Chinese medicine. (Ayu 7)

Nine of the fifteen interviewees reported this pattern. This order of events also influences the ways in which they use Ayurvedic medicine. These medical doctors are far from practising a purist form of Ayurveda. Instead, we can observe hybrid combinations with biomedical diagnostics or other forms of heterodox medicine. Sometimes Ayurvedic concepts are heavily merged with other approaches, so that new forms of medical practice emerge (Frank 2004).

Unease with biomedicine – technicalisation versus holism

These two motives – affinity with Indian culture, existing practice of heterodox medicine – can be complemented by further aspects. Again, we find critical attitudes towards biomedicine. While medical homoeopaths attacked the therapeutic effects of biomedical strategies, Ayurvedic physicians reject biomedical *philosophy*. They regard biomedicine as too technical and not patient-centred:

> It started at university when the mainstream increasingly drifted towards high-tech medicine. Everything became so over-the-top with the most expensive machines and the most incredible hygiene. I hated it. (Ayu 11)

> I decided to go for alternative medicine while I was already working. When I experienced the daily routine in hospital, I told myself: 'No, I do not want to practise like that.' Biomedicine is so mechanical and technical in the way that it deals with the body: Something is out of order and it has to be fixed by chemistry or surgery. (Ayu 5)

> It was caused by biomedicine. I used to work as a radiologist and became so frustrated with it. It is so hostile to the patients, so inhumane. I was working with MRT [Magnet Resonance Tomography – a diagnostic technique] where you push the patient through the pipe and that's it. Nobody even talks to the patient! (Ayu 9)

Contrary to the clinical, analytical approach used in biomedicine, the Ayurvedic physicians in our study perceive the possibility of using Ayurveda to achieve synthesis. Because Ayurveda involves a holistic approach, one can transcend the fragmentary aspects of biomedicine:

> What I didn't like about biomedicine was that you take the person's body apart. That part of the body is then treated. Everything else is ignored. I have always been in favour of holism and holism is an essential part of Ayurveda. (Ayu 3)

> I am just convinced that modern medicine dissects the human being and we desperately need something in addition. We have to take the whole person into account and this is the only way in which medicine can be satisfying for the physician as well as for the patient. (Ayu 13)

Positive experience

Finally, a number of participants in our study experienced Ayurveda's efficacy before practising themselves, even though this was not as common as for medical homoeopaths. Three of the fifteen physicians interviewed reported their personal experiences to be a significant part of their motivation to study Ayurveda:

> I fell seriously ill. While biomedicine was helpful for a while, I had to complement the treatment with other means to become healthier. Ayurveda worked really well in that respect. (Ayu 1)

Few physicians of Indian descent practise Ayurveda in Germany. Only three of the one hundred Ayurvedic physicians in Germany have family ties to

India. We can assume that they were led to Ayurveda along different paths from their German colleagues:

> Even though I grew up in Germany, I have a huge family in India. So whenever I was there and had the flu, they gave me Ayurvedic medicines. (Ayu 8)

However, only a few Ayurvedic physicians mention experiences that prompted their decision to turn to Ayurvedic practice. It is much more common for them to report their affinity with Indian culture or their existing heterodox focus. We will see whether we can find similar patterns for a much more popular form of Asian medicine: acupuncture.

Medical acupuncturists

Acupuncture and Ayurveda were both developed in Asia, but their standing in the German health care system is totally different. There are around two hundred times more medical acupuncturists than Ayurvedic physicians. Public health insurance companies are much more willing to reimburse for acupuncture than for Ayurveda.[11] Medical doctors practise acupuncture for very different reasons to those given by their Ayurvedic colleagues for practising Ayurveda, however the data on medical acupuncturists is not as clear as that on homoeopathic and Ayurvedic physicians. Critical attitudes towards biomedicine were displayed by two physicians, although their views were markedly milder than the views of homoeopathic and Ayurvedic physicians. One acupuncturist was interested in heterodox medicine before becoming aware of acupuncture. Interviewees also reported that their interest in acupuncture was triggered more by chance, e.g., 'a friend/colleague told me about it' or 'completely by accident'. Heterodox practice does not appear to be deeply rooted in their pasts and there is little indication that a turning point in their career was when they started practising acupuncture.

Economic considerations

When economic aspects of heterodox medical practice are discussed, it is usually done in a negative fashion. Public health insurance companies do not pay for non-biomedical modes of treatment in most countries and heterodox physicians earn significantly less than biomedical doctors (Goldstein et al. 1988). For the purist Ayurvedic physicians in our sample, who mainly focus on Ayurveda in their practice, this was particularly the case. None of them could make a living out of their Ayurvedic practice alone and needed another stream of income. In the case of acupuncture, things are different. Acupuncture's popularity continues to be high and it is the most commonly used form of heterodox medicine in many parts of the world. These aspects are reflected in some of the doctors' comments on their reasons for turning to acupuncture:

Anyone who intends to become a doctor these days has to take the financial aspect into account. There is no way around that. And acupuncture complements biomedicine well. I'm saving a lot of money on drug prescription. Economics are important nowadays, even though you also have to have a passion for acupuncture. Otherwise you will never be able to use it successfully. And I am also investing time and money in the training. (...) It is a chance to treat the patients comprehensively and – at the same time – a good source of income. What are the others telling you? (Acu[12] 8)

I took this practice over from a Persian physician who used acupuncture for many years. So when his patients kept coming, I thought: 'Why not learn acupuncture? The demand is there.' I have to admit that it was not until later on that I became increasingly fascinated by Chinese medicine. (Acu 9)

Acupuncture is one of the few forms of heterodox medicine that is reliably lucrative for practitioners. While the reasons for the remarkable success of acupuncture in 'Western' countries are beyond the scope of this paper, the social standing of acupuncture seems to influence the motivations of medical doctors. Only two of the fourteen physicians interviewed reported that economic considerations were important to them. Both of them were clearly hesitant to talk about this and their answers appeared to be minor confessions, as taking up acupuncture for (economic) self-interest is certainly not in line with medical ethics. However, the majority of interviewees knew of *other* doctors who had a strongly economical approach to acupuncture:

There is an increasing demand for this holistic approach among patients, so therefore more and more practitioners are offering acupuncture, because you can make a lot of money out of it nowadays. You have to say that very clearly. The whole boom in Germany started *after* the fees were rising. Many went for a few weekend workshops and see it as a way of making money. Those who are trying to work seriously with this method will be disadvantaged because acupuncture's reputation will suffer. Patients are already saying: 'My orthopaedist already tried out acupuncture. It didn't help'. (Acu 14)

Acupuncture has a strong presence in the media and is increasingly offered. That is rather a disadvantage, because a lot of low-quality acupuncture will inevitably harm the method. (Acu 6)

Not surprisingly, none of these 'selfish' physicians could be found in this sample. We can assume that the physicians were conscious of giving a socially desirable impression during the interview, which makes it difficult to assess the significance of economic factors. It would be no surprise if more than these two doctors had economic considerations in mind before choosing acupuncture as the heterodox mode of their liking. It is hard to decide whether the vagueness of medical acupuncturists' answers when questioned about their motives supports this interpretation.

Asian philosophy

Two of the fourteen physicians who participated in this study reported that their interest in acupuncture grew from their fascination in Asian culture. Again, trips to Asia initiated contact with foreign medical modes:

> Before I started studying, I travelled to India, Nepal and Thailand. And this trip really changed my approach to human life. I have been a vegetarian since then and I was so intrigued by the whole world of thought behind Chinese medicine. I felt closer to it than to homoeopathy, for example. (Acu 2)

> You see, in the early 1980s people became increasingly open to the East. Everything Asian became fascinating and you got hold of a book on it and then five books. Then you get hooked and you never stop. (Acu 10)

It is interesting that for both of these physicians, it doesn't appear to have been *Chinese* culture specifically that laid the foundation for their interest in acupuncture. Acupuncturist 2 has not travelled to China, but has travelled to other Asian countries. It was clear that these two physicians were merely interested in all things Asian.

There are a lot of open questions concerning the motives of medical acupuncturists, which cannot be answered by this study. It is interesting that the data did not necessarily reflect commonly held assumptions about the motives of heterodox medical doctors. For example, German medical acupuncturists did not have any harsh criticisms of either biomedical efficacy or its philosophy. Even personal experiences with acupuncture did not figure in their accounts of their professional history. It would also be reading too much into it to hold Chinese culture responsible for the physicians' interest in acupuncture.

Medical acupuncturists' practice is as varied as their motives. Acupuncture can represent between 1 per cent and 98 per cent of their overall treatment, and we can find purist approaches as well as various forms of hybrid ideas (Frank and Stollberg 2004).

Discussion

One of the purposes of this study was to test Goldstein's (1985) and Goldstein et al.'s (1988) results on medical doctors' motives for becoming heterodox physicians. However, only a few of them could be confirmed as being applicable to the German context. In particular, spiritual leanings and personal crises hardly figured in the physicians' accounts. This suggests that Goldstein's results might be limited either to the Californian or organisational context of the American Holistic Medical Association. Apart from regional factors, historical aspects could also be involved. Goldstein's data were collected in the early 1980s, while this study was conducted around the year 2000. During the nearly two decades in between, the standing of heterodox medicine has changed significantly. Heterodox medicine became increasingly popular among the public (Eisenberg et al. 1993) as well as the medical profession (Verhoef and Sunderland 1995, Tovey 1997). The increasing societal acceptance of heterodox medicine is most clearly reflected in two reports by the British Medical Association (BMA) on heterodox medicine (British Medical Association 1986, 1993). While the 1986 report is rather hostile, alleging that heterodox medicine is unscientific, the BMA adopts a completely different approach seven years later: Heterodox modes of treatment are now seen as potentially helpful strategies that are able to complement biomedical treatment. We can assume that the higher social standing of heterodox modes of medicine might give doctors different reasons to practise them (Cant and Sharma 1999). When we look at the data of this study it becomes evident that only Ayurvedic physicians show some resemblance to Goldstein's AHMA physicians. This is consistent with Ayurveda's current standing in the German health care system, which is about as marginal as heterodox medicine as a whole when Goldstein collected his data. Of the three groups in this study, German Ayurvedic physicians adopt the most philosophical and idealistic approach to being a medical doctor. A significant proportion of them does not even shy away from economic difficulties, which forces them to look for part-time jobs in order make ends meet.

Further research is required in order to determine the motives of all three groups of physicians. The most ambiguous data gathered relate to medical acupuncturists. How can this be explained? The same research methods were used for all three groups of medical doctors. Since comparatively rich data could be collected on homoeopathic and Ayurvedic physicians, it cannot be attributed to our questionnaire. It appears more likely that the vague accounts of medical acupuncturists were due to a major limitation associated with qualitative interviewing: the wish to give a socially desirable impression. While there are numerous *other* physicians – particularly orthopaedists and surgeons who take up acupuncture for monetary reasons, only two participants 'confessed' that economic considerations were relevant to their choice of acupuncture. One might suspect that these *other physicians* refused to take part in this study. However, 100 per cent of acupuncturists approached participated in the study. The vagueness of their answers raises the question: Were they *unwilling* or *unable* to provide more precise accounts of their motives? This is all idle speculation as there is no way of finding out what the interviewees might have been silent about. Saks' way of analysing the strategies of professional institutions (1992, 1994, 1995) is only moderately helpful, because individual physicians' attitudes can deviate from the approaches taken by their organisational bodies, as was shown for homoeopathy (Cant and Sharma 1996, Frank 2002b). Therefore, we have to distinguish between the practising physicians and the professional organisations of biomedicine as well as heterodox medicine. It appears impossible to identify any homogeneous approaches within *the* medical profession in dealing with heterodox medicine.

Additionally, our data suggest that professional self-interest is limited to the heterodox mode, which is – at least in contemporary Germany – the most lucrative: acupuncture. While hypotheses based on professionalisation theory can provide important insights, it is preferable to resort to empirical studies. As regards the problem involving the vague answers given by medical acupuncturists, research structured a different way may achieve more reliable results: Quantitative studies might be able to provide a more anonymous environment in which social desirability has less influence on the answers than in face-to-face interviews. Survey studies could also be beneficial for examining the other groups of this study, as they would enable the relative importance of the respective motives to be assessed.

There are no signs that heterodox medical doctors perceive themselves as the heretics described by Wolpe (1990) and Dew (1997). None of the forty-nine interviewees reported being persecuted or disciplined by biomedical organisations.[13] However, antagonism between heterodox medical doctors and the biomedical world varies between the three groups of physicians in our study. Interestingly enough, the most fundamental criticism was not mounted by physicians who practise the most marginalised system (Ayurveda), but by doctors using a heterodox mode that is well established in Germany for a long time: homoeopathy. Homoeopathic concepts appear to be partly responsible for this antagonism. It is particularly difficult to reconcile homoeopathic strategies with biomedical ones (Frank 2002b). The most central concept in homoeopathy – similia similibus curentur ('like cures like') – is in sharp contrast with biomedical concepts, which have been coined allopathy by homoeopaths for this reason. Therefore, conflicts between biomedical and homoeopathic physicians have been particularly fierce during the last two centuries. This hostility is consistent with the reported motives of homoeopathic physicians. For them, disillusionment with biomedical practice is particularly strong, while on the other hand, Ayurvedic physicians appear to be drawn to Ayurveda due to its connection with Indian culture or their heterodox orientation. Even though data on medical acupuncturists were vague, it can be assumed that the attractions – be they of an economic nature or not – are more relevant to them than alienation from biomedicine.

Despite its limitations, the presented study is able to offer new insights into the motives of heterodox medical doctors. The most important message might be to point out the differences between the three groups of physicians. It is not possible to identify one homogenous motivational pattern for heterodox medical doctors. This would have been surprising given that heterodox medicine is a broad field. This study cannot clarify the relative importance of the ontologies of the respective modes of treatment and their social standing, which contribute to their appeal to physicians. An international comparison with other health care systems in which the standing of homoeopathy, acupuncture and Ayurveda is different might shed light on this critical issue and enable us to increase our knowledge of the processes that lead medical doctors to practise heterodox medicine.

Notes

1. The Maharishi Ayurveda organisation manages health centres, a network of physicians, Ayurvedic training as well as the distribution of Ayurvedic drugs.
2. www.ayurveda-gesellschaft.de
3. 90 per cent of the German population has public health insurance. Private health insurance is only open to self-employed people or those who enjoy a higher income. Therefore, the reimbursement policies of public health insurance companies have a great impact on the standing of heterodox medicine in Germany.
4. 'Hom' stands for homoeopath.
5. The principle of *similia similibus curentur* ('like cures like') is the central strategy in homoeopathic healing. It means that homoeopathic remedies should produce the very symptoms in a healthy human being that they eliminate when applied to a person with a particular disease. Remedies are described in terms of symptoms, which should resemble the patient's symptoms as much as possible.
6. While this institutional category is specific to the German health care system, it is comparable to 'lay practitioners' elsewhere. The practice of *Heilpraktiker* is based on legislation passed by the Nazi regime in 1935 that tried to regulate the practice of 'lay practitioners'. Applicants have to pass an exam in subjects such as anatomy, physiology and pathology. Once they pass these tests, they are free to practice whatever medical tradition they please. Without the qualification, the professional treatment of patients is illegal in Germany.
7. 'Ayu' stands for Ayurvedic physician.
8. Heinrich Harrer became famous for his novel 'Seven Years in Tibet'.
9. Authoritative Ayurvedic textbooks.
10. Medical homoeopaths in Germany either segregated their patients into two categories, namely homoeopathic or biomedical patients, complemented a predominantly homoeopathic practice with a few biomedical strategies for diagnostics, or focused on homoeopathy and condemned biomedicine.
11. At present, each patient has to apply for acupuncture. In cases of chronic pain (migraine, back pain), patients' requests are usually approved and full reimbursement is provided. In other cases, health insurance companies offer only limited support.
12. 'Acu' stands for acupuncturist.
13. Medical doctors must be members of the main organisational body for doctors (*Bundesärztekammer*).

References

British Medical Association. 1986. *Alternative Therapy Report of the Board of Science and Education*. London: British Medical Association.
—— 1993. *Complementary Medicine. New Approaches to Good Practice*. Oxford: British Medical Association.
Cant, S. and U. Sharma. 1996. 'Demarcation and Transformation within Homoeopathic Knowledge. A Strategy of Professionalisation', *Social Science & Medicine* 42: 579–588.
—— 1999. *A New Medical Pluralism? Alternative Medicine, Doctors, Patients and the State*. London: Routledge.
Dew, K. 1997. 'Limits on the Utilization of Alternative Therapies by Doctors in New Zealand: A Problem of Boundary Maintenance', *Australian Journal of Social Issues* 32: 181–196.

Eisenberg, D., R. Kessler, C. Foster, F. Norlock, D. Calkins and T. Delbanco. 1993. 'Unconventional Medicine in the United States', *New England Journal of Medicine* 328: 246–252.

Fairclough, N. (1992) *Discourse and Social Change.* Cambridge: Polity.

Frank, R. 2002a. 'Homoeopath and Patient – a Dyad of Harmony? Patterns of Communication, Sources of Conflict and Expectations in Homoeopathic Physician-patient-relationship', *Social Science & Medicine* 55: 1285–1296.

——2002b. 'Integrating Homoeopathy and Biomedicine. Medical Practice and Knowledge Production among German Homoeopathic Physicians', *Sociology of Health and Illness* 24: 796–819.

——2004. *Globalisierung 'alternativer' Medizin. Homoeopathie und Ayurveda in Deutschland und Indien.* Bielefeld: Transcript.

Frank, R. and G. Stollberg. 2002. 'Ayurvedic Patients in Germany', *Anthropology & Medicine* 9: 223–244.

——2004. 'Conceptualising Hybridisation – on the Diffusion of Asian Medical Knowledge to Germany', *International Sociology* 19(1): 71–88.

Furnham, A. and C. Smith. 1988. 'Choosing Alternative Medicine: a Comparison of the Beliefs of Patients Visiting a General Practitioner and a Homoeopath', *Social Science & Medicine* 26: 685–689.

Goldstein, M.S. 1985. 'Holistic Doctors. Becoming a Nontraditional Medical Practitioner', *Urban Life,* 14: 317–344.

Goldstein, M.S., C. Sutherland, D.T. Jaffe and J. Wilson. 1988. 'Holistic Physicians and Family Practitioners: Similarities, Differences and Implications for Health Policy', *Social Science & Medicine* 26: 853–861.

Lynöe, N. and T. Svensson. 1992. 'Physicians and Alternative Medicine: an Investigation of Attitudes and Practice', *Scandinavian Journal of Medicine,* 20: 55–60.

Mayring, P. 1988. *Qualitative Inhaltsanalyse.* Weinheim: Deutscher Studien Verlag.

Saks, M. 1992. 'The Paradox of Incorporation: Acupuncture and the Medical Profession in Britain', in M. Saks (ed.) *Alternative Medicine in Britain.* Oxford: Clarendon Press, 183–200.

——1994. 'The Alternatives to Medicine', in J. Gabe, D. Kelleher and G. Williams (eds) *Challenging Medicine.* London: Routledge, 84–102.

——1995. 'The Changing Response of the Medical Profession to Alternative Medicine in Britain: a Case of Self-interest or Altruism', in T. Johnson, G. Larkin and M. Saks (eds) *The Health Professions and the State in Europe.* London: Routledge, 103–115.

Sharma, U. 1990. 'Using Alternative Therapies: Marginal Medicine and Central Concerns', in P. Abbot and G. Payne (eds) *New Directions in the Sociology of Health,* London: Falmer Press, 127–139.

——1992. *Complementary Medicine Today.* London: Routledge.

Stollberg, G. 2001. *Medizinsoziologie.* Bielefeld: Transcript.

——2002. 'Patients and Homoeopathy: an Overview of Sociological Literature', in M. Dinges (ed.) *Patients in the History of Homoeopathy.* Sheffield: EAHMH Publications, 317–329.

Sudman, S., N.M. Bradburn and N. Schwarz. 1996. *Thinking about Answers: the Application of Cognitive Processes to Survey Methodology.* San Francisco: Jossey-Bass.

Tovey, P. 1997. 'Contingent Legitimacy: UK Alternative Practitioners and Inter-sectorial Acceptance', *Social Science & Medicine,* 45: 1129–1133.

Verhoef, M.J. and L.R. Sutherland. 1995. '"General Practitioners" Assessment of and Interest in Alternative Treatment in Canada', *Social Science & Medicine* 41: 511–515.

Wolpe, P.R. 1990. 'The Holistic Heresy: Strategies of Ideological Challenge in the Medical Profession', *Social Science & Medicine* 31: 913–923.

6

Pluralisms of Provision, Use and Ideology
Homoeopathy in South London

Christine A. Barry

Homoeopathy represents an interesting case of pluralism of healthcare provision. It was one of the earlier of the currently popular alternative therapies to arrive in the United Kingdom in the early nineteenth century (Porter 1997). It became one of the earliest of the modern alternative therapies to be offered by orthodox physicians and integrated into the orthodox health care system. Homoeopathy was incorporated into the National Health Service (NHS) at its inception in 1947, becoming the first of the alternative therapies to be offered in tandem with orthodox healthcare services in the NHS (Nicholls 1992).

Homoeopathy arrived in Britain shortly after it had been established in the early 1800s by a German physician, Samuel Hahnemann. Hahnemann developed a new system of medicine based on the principle of treating like with like. He discovered this 'law of similars' when he ingested the bark of the Chinchona tree (Quinine) and experienced a fever similar to malarial symptoms. He went on to chart the action of a wide variety of substances through 'proving' (testing) them on healthy people. The classical homoeopathy that he developed involves trying to match the overall picture of a person's symptoms to the remedy that itself produces the most similar pattern of symptoms in the healthy.

Dr Quin brought homoeopathy to England in 1828. It quickly evolved into two distinct forms of homoeopathy, each operating according to different principles and practiced by groups of homoeopaths with different training and philosophical principles.

Dr Quin was medically trained. He set up the British Homoeopathic Society which restricted membership to doctors and was rooted in reactionary political principles. It was a hierarchical, elitist organisation modelled on the Royal Colleges of Surgeons and Physicians. Hahnemann's ideas were tempered by integrating them with medical ideas and downplaying spiritual elements. Quin went on to found the London Homoeopathic Hospital in 1849.

In tandem with the development of the medical version of homoeopathy was the growth of the lay form of homoeopathy. The English Homoeopathy Association was set up in the 1830s as a reaction against the elitist, exclusionary strategy of the medical homoeopaths. It offered a more radical view of homoeopathy, encouraged practice by non-medically trained people and involved patients more. This model of homoeopathy was closer to Hahnemann's intended doctrine: it disregarded diseases and paid attention to the unique picture of individuals' symptoms, including those that might seem trivial to medical practitioners. It also maintained the spiritual dimension.

Both versions of homoeopathy are alive and well today. Contemporary British patients have the right to request referral for homoeopathic treatment on the NHS. Around nine hundred doctors have some training in homoeopathy, many work within the five homoeopathic hospitals and a number incorporate homoeopathy into their work as general practitioners.

There are also currently over four hundred fully trained professional homoeopaths in the United Kingdom represented by lay homoeopathy associations such as The Society of Homoeopaths, the majority practice privately. The provision of homoeopathy in the United Kingdom can therefore be seen as inherently pluralistic since its inception. The plurality relates to the training of therapists: medical versus lay; the philosophical underpinnings of the therapy: biomedicalised versus a more spiritual and holistic version; and the location of provision: inside the NHS medical system and outside (community based projects and private practice). This is not a simple dualism of provision as there are lay homoeopaths practising in NHS settings (e.g., Treuherz 1999) and many medical homoeopaths have left general practice to provide classical homoeopathy privately (Thompson et al. 2002).

Integration: a new medical pluralism

Homoeopathy's inclusion in NHS settings is part of a trend towards integration of all sorts of alternative medicines into the NHS (Zollman and Vickers 1999). The current United Kingdom system of health provision encourages 'A New Medical Pluralism' (Cant and Sharma 1999). Many members of the public are now coming to alternative medicine directly through the interventions of biomedical doctors who are either offering alternative techniques themselves or are referring to alternative therapists outside the health service (Thomas et al. 2003). This might not therefore require active seeking for alternative solutions, as in societies where alternatives are external to biomedicine. Traditional anthropological studies of pluralism have tended to focus on the patients, carers and families as active seekers of healthcare, looking for answers to unresolved healthcare problems, navigating their way through different healing systems. See for example Amarasingham's (1980) case study in Sri Lanka and more recently Lindquist's (2002) in Russia.

Where alternatives are offered within biomedical national health systems there is evidence for syncretism between biomedical and alternative practices. For example Dew (2000) details biomedical acupuncturists in New Zealand as having appropriated aspects of acupuncture into their biomedical practice. In the recent British House of Lords report on Complementary and Alternative Medicine, the separation out of medical acupuncture from Traditional Chinese Medicine, as more suitable for integration into the biomedical system shows the same tendencies towards dissecting, medicalising and syncretising alternative systems to fit biomedical philosophies and practices (House of Lords Select Committee on Science and Technology 2000).

The biomedical system has thus paradoxically become an agent of promotion of medical pluralism. In place of active consumers navigating multiple health systems, we now have active providers offering multiple solutions under one roof; sometimes to passive patients not actively seeking alternatives. The clear divide between biomedicine and alternative medicine has become blurred.

Current use of homoeopathy in the United Kingdom

A recent survey found 20 per cent of the UK population had used an alternative therapy in the last year, the most common being homoeopathy, herbal medicine and aromatherapy (Ernst and White 2000). Users are most likely to be women (24 per cent), between 35–64 years old (26 per cent) and in higher socio-economic groups AB (25 per cent).

In addition to the provision of homoeopathy by different sorts of practitioner there is also the option of self-medication without recourse to any practitioner. Homoeopathic remedies are freely available in many general pharmacies (See Figure 6.1). There are also manuals aimed at self-medication of acute minor health problems (e.g., Castro 1995). A recent survey found that 9 per cent of a UK sample had used an over-the-counter homoeopathic remedy in the past year, and 15 per cent in their lives (Thomas et al. 2001). Only 1 per cent claimed to have visited a homoeopath in the past twelve months, and 6 per cent in their lives. This survey did not differentiate between consultation of medical and professional homoeopaths.

There are no exact figures for the use of homoeopathy in primary care but a recent survey of general practice, showed that one in two practices in England now offer their patients access to alternative medicines by either providing them in-house or via referrals (Thomas et al. 2003).

Homoeopathy in South London

Having set the scene, historically and statistically, I now want to present data on contemporary pluralism in homoeopathy collected for my doctorate. This comprised a multi-site ethnography conducted 2000–2001 in a number of homoeopathy related settings in South London (Barry 2003).

Research method

The sites were chosen to represent different arenas of interaction: the clinical practice of homoeopathy, inside and outside the NHS, and other relevant interactions outside the clinic in community projects and educational settings. I represented medical and professional practitioners. The sites were as follows:

1. *A one-year 'Introduction to Homoeopathy' course*, at an adult education college, taught by a professional homoeopath. I attended weekly half-day seminars for a year, and attended informal meetings arranged at group members' houses. Ten students completed an open-ended questionnaire and I interviewed four in depth at home.
2. *A Vaccination Support Group* run by two professional homoeopaths, for parents deciding whether to vaccinate their children, and investigating alternative homoeopathic treatment strategies. This was held in the home of a group member. I attended monthly meetings for eighteen months, interviewed the facilitators and six attenders.
3. *A low cost homoeopathy clinic* in a Victim Support Centre, for victims of violent crime, run by two professional homoeopaths. I observed seven clinics over a six month period. With consent, I tape-recorded twenty-three consultations and interviewed six users.
4. *An NHS general practice* in which one of the doctors was a medical homoeopath. I observed his surgeries over a three month period, tape-recorded twenty-three consultations, and interviewed the senior partner, practice manager, receptionists and seven patients.
5. I also consulted with three professional homoeopaths as a patient to experience embodied issues of homoeopathy use. I visited one twice; consulted a second for six months; and a third for a year. I consulted monthly. They all agreed to see me knowing this would inform my research. I interviewed two about their treatment strategy and about their practice.
6. I also interviewed a professional homoeopath who worked part-time in general practice and four general practitioners (GPs) who worked alongside homoeopaths.

I had differing levels and nature of participation in the sites I researched. I was present as an embodied patient in my own consultations and so learned about homoeopathy through thoughts and feelings in consultations and bodily responses to treatment as a patient. I participated as an active learner in the adult education class: completing homework and reading, and taking part in seminar discussions. In the other sites I was more of an observer. My participation drew me into a more alternative view of health than I had held before fieldwork; which I then found retreated somewhat after fieldwork (Barry 2002).

The different sites allowed me to investigate different aspects of homoeopathy. The education class showed some people's views of health changing, while others resisted. In the vaccination group I saw how groups of people discussed homoeopathy and mutually constructed notions of health and healthcare, and methods of resistance to biomedical dominance. Interviews with GPs and homoeopaths gave me insight into the cosmology of the practitioners. Observations of consultations revealed how homoeopathy was played out in clinical interaction. Interviews with patients revealed how views and beliefs affected experiences of the consultation.

Medical pluralism in use and provision of homoeopathy in South London

I want to demonstrate two variants of pluralism with respect to the use of homoeopathy in South London. The first of these is a pluralism of healthcare-seeking behaviour which results in patients pursuing alternative healthcare provision to that offered by the state supported biomedical system. The second pluralism relates to the pluralistic provision of a number of different systems of healthcare within the state biomedical system, with different systems of healing offered by individual healthcare providers.

All homoeopathy users in my study continue to use orthodox medical services, representing pluralistic use of healthcare systems. However for some, beliefs about health and healing change over time, and this alters the ways in which they use orthodox services. The group I call 'committed users' come to hold a holistic, homoeopathic ideology of health. They see homoeopathy as a comprehensive alternative system, far preferable to orthodox medicine. They reduce dealings with the orthodox system to a minimum. This group actively sought alternative healthcare, usually outside the biomedical system. The second group, 'pragmatic users', maintain a more biomedical ideology. They use homoeopathy on occasion, but view it as an inferior complement to orthodox medicine. So while both use pluralistic health systems they do so in different ways.

To some extent this dual model of pluralism arises from the dualistic model of homoeopathy provision outlined in the preceding review of homoeopathy's history. The pragmatic users came to homoeopathy without actively seeking it out. Some happened upon a homoeopathic GP in their local NHS general practice.

Committed users: actively seeking alternatives

In the view of those committed users who see homoeopathy as an alternative, health is not a property of individuals but of interconnected systems which encompass people in relationships with each other and with the environment. Illness is a positive part of health and occurs across a mind-body-spirit unity.

All seventeen committed users sought out homoeopathic treatment having found biomedicine wanting. All but four consult a private homoeopath regularly. They are sufficiently committed to pay private rates. Their view of health, illness and treatment is quite different from the biomedical view, and similar to the views of their non-medical practitioners. Six main beliefs about health, illness and healing are commonly voiced:

1. Health is an ongoing interdependent relationship with the social, physical and spiritual environment. Emotions and relationships are primary catalysts for illness.
2. Illness and symptoms are an active, positive part of health.
3. The healing process starts with health not sickness.
4. The body is the active, natural agent of healing.
5. Homoeopathy assists the body: orthodox drugs suppress symptoms and hinder healing.
6. The user has primary responsibility for healthcare; resulting in more egalitarian relationships with healthcare providers.

The users come to espouse these views in a very committed and enthusiastic way. Their adherence to this belief system could be seen in terms of a conversion to a new religion. Homoeopathy offers more than just treatment for health problems. It appears to appeal at a deeper level of spiritual need, providing answers to questions of meaning, through a framework in which to make sense of their lives.

In spite of the fervour of their new views they do not leave behind the orthodox healthcare system. They all continue to interact with this system, but reject many aspects of medical care. Jean, a user and student explains:

[Homoeopathy is] a safe and pleasant way to aid the body to restore its own good health without the use of blanket drugs with long-term or short-term side-effects. I would like to think that in the case of a major disease affecting one of us we could use [homoeopathic] remedies to help us deal psychologically with the problem as well as physically. I very rarely visit the doctor at all.

An opposition to orthodox medicine is inherent within this version of homoeopathic cosmology. Committed users resist drugs and refuse vaccinations. They report disappointment with the lack of attention within medical consultations to social lifeworld issues, such as bereavement and relationship difficulties. In prior research I have explored this tendency of general practice consultations to suppress patients agendas and ignore the voice of the lifeworld (Barry et al. 2000, 2001).

This use of two medical systems in tandem has been documented (Cant and Sharma 1999) but not how use of the orthodox system changes. Among the committed users there is a universal experience of interacting differently:

1. The homoeopath replaces the function of a GP as primary healthcare provider.
2. Many report using GPs purely for diagnoses and tests. Some would only use them for acute emergencies or surgery.
3. They assertively resist proposed biomedical interventions.
4. Some actively seek out homoeopathic GPs in addition to their homoeopaths for consistency of philosophy across healthcare providers.

Ruth: a committed homoeopathy user

Ruth exemplifies several of these changes. She is forty-two, a student, with a five-year old daughter Lily, for whom she shares childcare with her ex-partner Tim. Ruth has been pluralistic in her healthcare seeking for twenty years and uses a range of alternative therapies. She first consulted aged nineteen after a miscarriage, with a bad back. She visited osteopaths, chiropractors and physiotherapists, and still visits an osteopath whenever it flares up. At thirty Ruth was diagnosed with cancer. She wanted to visit the Bristol Cancer Help Centre but could not afford to. However she was inspired by advice in their book about diet and alternatives, and sought out a naturopath. Part of her justification was needing control:

> I felt like I was totally out of control of this thing that had invaded my body and if I'd left it to the hands of the medical profession I wouldn't have been playing a very active role in my treatment at all.

A year later Ruth feared a brain tumour signalling the return of her cancer (it turned out to be an inner ear infection). She felt very angry and let down by the naturopath, when he did not return her calls for a week, and stopped visiting him. A friend recommended a homoeopath who she has visited regularly for the past eleven years. When baby Lily had severe colic Ruth was told by her doctor she would just have to live with it. She took Lily to a cranial osteopath who cured her after two sessions. Ruth takes Lily to the homoeopath for ongoing care. Ruth is working part time to support her studies and is on a low income. She told me she had spent 'an absolute fortune but it is worth it', because she believes in it. Ruth continues to visit her homoeopath monthly and rarely thinks about her cancer. Recent visits focus on her depression since the split with her partner.

A number of factors have been implicated in Ruth's pluralistic healthcare-seeking strategies. In part she has selected therapies to suit her particular health problem: osteopathy for back problems, naturopathy for her cancer, cranial osteopathy for Lily's colic. Homoeopathy has come to be her main therapy in part as a result of the very trusting relationship with her homoeopath.

Interacting with different therapists makes Ruth feel more in control. She makes informed decisions about which to consult and keeps each of her therapists informed. She tells her homoeopath, Jenny, that her osteopath reported at the last session 'there's no feeling between your head and your womb'. Jenny gets Ruth talking about her early miscarriage and treats her homoeopathically for the after-effects of this.

> Jenny is very happy for me to see other alternative practitioners. The way I work it is that I let each of them know, what's going on with the other one so that they can each put a whole picture together... That's what I do with my osteopath as well. She's often interested in what remedies I'm having from Jenny. So we, sort of, work in a triangular way, with me being the main person.

Ruth's changed use of the orthodox medical system

Ruth positions her homoeopath as primary healthcare provider, other alternative therapists, such as her osteopath, as supplementary specialists, with her GP purely as a route to hospital specialists:

> Sometimes [GPs] are quite useful if you need a referral. That's when I try to use them. But now that I'm feeling much more knowledgeable about the homoeopathy I will try homoeopathy first and ring Jenny. Homoeopathy is the first port of call and then if it gets really serious or doesn't change I'll then go to the doctor, either for confirmation or a second opinion. I don't like going.

Ruth reports feeling 'empowered' by her interactions with alternative medicine. The homoeopathic explanations for her illness make more intuitive sense and the fact her therapists share their knowledge makes her feel responsible for her health in a way that she hasn't felt with orthodox medicine:

> On the one hand the [oncology doctors] are saying 'oh you can't do this' and 'you mustn't have a baby' and 'you must do that'. But actually in the same breath they are saying, 'we don't know what is wrong with you really. We can't tell you what type of cancer it is. We can't answer any of your questions'. They are very definite about one thing but not another, and I just feel that those two don't marry up. On the other hand I've got the homoeopath and the osteopaths looking at the whole picture, both as I present it now and historically, and my family; and saying 'OK where's this cancer come from?' One homoeopath talked about it being an emotional blockage in my system, a blockage of anger which has just manifested

itself as a tumour. I thought 'Mm that makes sense to me' in a way that was so completely different from what the medical profession were telling me. And it gave me hope. It really did give me hope.

Through her use of alternatives she has developed a negative attitude to biomedical drugs, vaccinations and interventions: 'When I had my bad back [twenty years ago] I had a cortisone injection into the muscle. Well I wouldn't dream of doing that now'. Lily has not had any vaccinations, and Ruth attended the vaccination group for a year when Lily was a baby.

It would appear to be biomedical treatment that she is mostly against, rather than the personnel as she told me she would really love it if she could find a homoeopathic GP: 'Then you're getting the best of both worlds'. There is one locally but his books are full. Interestingly, committed users like Ruth are more enthusiastic about homoeopathic GPs in theory than in practice.

Seeking alternative homoeopathy philosophy from a homoeopathic GP

In another setting Helen, one of the students of homoeopathy, reports her excitement to the adult education class about getting an appointment with a homoeopathic GP. By chance it is Dr Deakin with whom I am about to start fieldwork. As an impoverished single mother she has high hopes, of getting the type of homoeopathic treatment we are learning about on the course via the NHS. She heads off very excited about the possibilities of homoeopathic treatment for her emotional problems, caused by the recent break up of her marriage. The course has also put the idea in her head that homoeopathic remedies have the capacity to heal long entrenched problems from the past and she hopes for a cure for leg pain she has suffered for eight years.

She is desolated after her visit. She tells me she did not get a chance to air any of her own problems; only her daughter's rash. She complains he had no time for her and seemed rather grumpy. She reports with amazement and disappointment: 'He was just like any other GP! He looked at me as if to say what are you doing here, wasting my time'. She vows never to go back to him. Later in the year she starts visiting a private homoeopath. Implicit in Helen's disappointment was the expectation of a very different kind of consultation and of homoeopathy as a unitary medical system, unaffected by provider or context.

Users who have come to homoeopathy via private homoeopathic services with non-medical homoeopaths, imagine a homoeopathic GP will operate in similar ways to their private homoeopath. They are not aware that NHS settings are very constraining on homoeopathic practice. Dr Deakin is different to the average GP, a gentle man, his patients say he 'has healing hands' is more 'human and humane' than other doctors, but he is still constrained by the NHS setting within which he works. For example, being expected to limit his consultations to an average of ten minutes. On the day of Helen's visit he was likely to be overworked and stressed. I saw him do 9.00am–8.00pm days with no break.

These users who welcome homoeopathy in general practice also may not be aware that medical homoeopaths are trained differently and are more likely to offer a more medicalised version of homoeopathy, paying more attention to physical symptoms. I have elaborated on these aspects of medical homoeopathy at greater length in my thesis (Barry 2003). This view is also emerging from the research of Trevor Thompson with medical homoeopaths in general practice (Thompson et al. 2002).

Pragmatic homoeopathy users: happening upon alternatives by chance

The second group of users in my study are also engaged in pluralistic healthcare strategies. However this is not self-initiated, but instigated by their providers of healthcare. They happen upon homoeopathy accidentally. I have called the ten people in my study who came to homoeopathy in this way Pragmatic Users.

They were initiated into homoeopathy via one of two routes. Those attending the victim support clinic as victims of recent crimes such as violent muggings, were surprised to find they were offered, in addition to practical help or counselling, the opportunity to consult with a professional homoeopath. As most were in vulnerable states: suffering from depression, grief, panic or sleeplessness, they were keen to get whatever help they could, even though most knew nothing about homoeopathy.

The other route was through attending the local general practice where Dr Deakin (mentioned above in conjunction with Helen's disappointed visit) offers several alternative therapies, including homoeopathy, alongside orthodox care. However patients are often unaware of this until he suggests a homoeopathic remedy in a consultation. The general practice is like any other and there is no indication in the waiting or reception areas that Dr Deakin is any different to the other three GPs in the practice. These patients are surprised by homoeopathy, but some are willing to 'give it a go'. Their pluralism is initiated by the pluralistic provision of their primary healthcare provider, not by themselves.

Joanne, Dr Deakin's patient, illustrates her view of homoeopathy:

[Homoeopathy] hasn't been proven, it's not been accepted, but eventually the two medicines will work together, homoeopathy as a complement to medicine. The choice [being] which of these two medicines is suitable for this particular complaint... If you've got cancer, don't kid yourself... As much as I have a belief in homoeopathic medicine, if you're in pain and/or you're really worried about something that has an obvious root cause, I wouldn't have the confidence to go along that course.

Fifty-eight year-old Joanne, a retired publican, lives in an exclusive large detached house in a leafy London suburb. When Joanne had breast cancer a few years ago she did not use alternative medicine nor has she at any other time in her life until she started seeing Dr Deakin. Her husband Charles is currently having radiotherapy for cancer, he hasn't tried alternatives. 'If somebody came along to me now and said, "If he drank this... it's homoeopathic, and it's for cancer" I'd encourage him to do it, but I've never even heard, in that particular field, of any doctor who practises that'. This implies that she would only consider alternative therapy if sanctioned by and provided by biomedical doctors, and specifically suitable for a biomedical diagnosis. General practice patients commonly express reluctance to use any medical treatment not sanctioned by their doctor (Stevenson et al. 2003).

Joanne has great respect for consultants for saving her granddaughter's life from an asthma attack and her own from cancer. 'My specialist, to me was my god, I mean I respect him, I respect his position, and I respect the medical profession... I have faith in the proven medicines of the hospital.' She stresses the scientific and advanced basis of biomedicine compared with homoeopathy.

At Dr Deakin's suggestion Joanne has used homoeopathic treatment to combat a recurrent chest infection. She reports her use with little enthusiasm, even though her infection was cured after this treatment. She is mainly using homoeopathy because she trusts the authority of her doctors:

> In my weak state he said, 'Now what do you want, do you want me to give you antibiotics or would you try the homoeopathic approach?' So I said, 'Well you're the doctor, you tell me.'

In a consultation I observed where Joanne had a swollen eyelid, Dr Deakin gave her the option of homoeopathic medicine:

> Dr Deakin: 'The options are: you can take a homoeopathic medicine if you feel happy with that. That has the least side effects. If you take anti-histamines they work in a similar way but make you a bit drowsy if you have to drive a car or something, but that would be the more chemical option. Or I can give you herbs?'
>
> Joanne: 'I'd like a quick reaction as opposed to a (inaudible – Dr saying OK) I'd rather take the... I think it's called the easy way out isn't it?'

So whilst Joanne has used homoeopathy at the suggestion of her doctor she is not buying into the homoeopathic model with enthusiasm. She told me: 'Dr Deakin comes over as being a much more caring man, but the fact that he leans immediately towards homoeopathy would stop me from seeing him all the time.' Joanne chooses orthodox medicine primarily and tries homoeopathy occasionally. Ideologically she remains very much in the biomedical model of illness and healing.

Laura, a visitor to the victim support centre homoeopathy clinic, is similar in many ways. Laura was mugged at night in a street near her home and is now terrified to go out. She visits Jenny the professional homoeopath once a fortnight over the first few months after the attack, and takes the homoeopathic remedies Jenny gives her. However she reports mainly valuing the 'talking cure' aspect of the therapy. 'There definitely is a place for talking therapy which I think is wonderful, I think everybody should have it.' Like Joanne she too has very positive beliefs about the orthodox medical system as 'a God-given thing' and voices doubts about alternatives in general, 'I think I've always been a little, not *anti* – but I'm glad they call it *complementary* medicine not alternative, now that was a good change'. She admits there may be a role for homoeopathy:

> There is another side of life that's not fully explored, and maybe that is where homoeopathy can step in. So I think I feel very ambivalent about it… I can't say to you it has solved this problem. I can't honestly say that. It may have been helpful, I can't tell.

There was no evidence at the time of my fieldwork, to suggest patients like Joanne or Laura are open to taking on different beliefs about health, healing and the body.

Pluralism of provision

The users in my study seem to have a fairly coherent and consistent set of beliefs about health and healing, whether it be the alternative beliefs of the committed users or the normative biomedical beliefs of the pragmatic users. The professional homoeopaths who share the alternative views of the committed users seem to share their consistent and singular belief system, although they also offer some pluralistic practice: Jenny uses Flower Essences alongside her homoeopathy, Eve practices Reiki and Nancy is training in sacro-cranial therapy.

Dr Deakin does not appear to share this singular health belief system. His practice suggests an element of biomedicalisation of homoeopathic principles. When he talks of holism it is a holism of body systems and does not extend out into the social relations and emotions so often discussed in non-medical homoeopathy consultations. I assume he is reflecting the medicalised version of homoeopathy as brought to the United Kingdom by Dr Quin and promoted through medical training courses.

In place of one clear-cut belief system, Dr Deakin appears to be working with multiple ideologies as well as practices. Where his NHS patients want orthodox medicine he offers conventional consultations; when they are open to alternatives he pursues different therapeutic options. In this sense he is like the first group of German homoeopathic doctors in Robert Frank's study (Frank, this volume). Frank suggests this group of doctors find it difficult to develop a professional identity. Dr Deakin appears to operate on various different identities. In his alternative consultations he draws on multiple possible treatment options for his patients; he employs diagnoses from different ideological approaches; and offers multiple explanations for treatment, often within the same consultation. In comparison with the non-medical homoeopaths he voices a more pluralistic and varied ideology fusing concepts from biomedicine, Chinese medicine and homoeopathy. This plurality manifests itself in his consultation behaviour.

In one surgery I observe Paul consulting Dr Deakin about his swollen eyelid. Paul enquires about possible homoeopathic and herbal remedies. Dr Deakin starts by suggesting herbal eyedrops, and then goes on to explain:

> In Chinese medicine, the upper eyelid relates to the liver, some sort of congestion, a toxic congestion of the liver, and the lower eyelid relates more to the kidney system, the genital-urinary system, and is more a sort of the bags of exhaustion. Western medicine hasn't quite accepted that view.

When Paul replies laughing (suggesting that he is surprised by this non sequitur), 'So should I do something about my liver rather than my eye?' Dr Deakin responds:

> Well... sounds like it (laughing). But that's Oriental medicine, we haven't made a proper Oriental diagnosis, so I very much try to keep to the homoeopathic treatment approach [therefore I will prescribe] *Euphrasia* eye drops.

This interchange shows that Dr Deakin is pluralistic, not only in his choice of treatment strategies, but in his choice of diagnoses. Dr Deakin is unlike the GP mentioned in Adams' and Tovey's (2000: 176) research, who said: 'You cannot sit here and see the patients for ten-minute intervals doing Western medicine and then switch for two minutes into Chinese medicine'. Dr Deakin does manage to do a bit of Western medicine, Chinese diagnosis and homoeopathic prescribing, within his general practice consultations.

In this sense Dr Deakin is similar to his more orthodox general practice colleagues. General practice is the most eclectic of medical specialities and spans a range of therapeutic options rooted in very different philosophical approaches: from minor surgery to counselling. GPs are used to switching between these at ten-minute intervals as a varied range of patients arrive in their surgeries. Perhaps the only difference with Dr Deakin is breadth of range of his therapeutic options.

Two different kinds of pluralism?

Through my data I hope I have demonstrated the effects of the historical pluralism of homoeopathic provision in the healthcare system in this country. As a result of homoeopathy being available inside the NHS in a more medicalised form, and outside, in a more ideologically separate system of healthcare, we have plural use of homoeopathy and orthodox medicine manifesting in quite different beliefs and behaviour for different groups of users.

The pluralistic nature of homoeopathy provision, as outlined earlier in the paper, is not really understood by many of the people I did research with. The general assumption is that homoeopathy is the same wherever it is practiced until people have some personal experience. The only people aware of their right to access homoeopathic treatment through the NHS were the two committed users who were, unusually, using Dr Deakin as their sole homoeopathy provider. Those solely consulting with private homoeopaths were not conscious of the differences with homoeopathy from the doctor. As we saw with Helen and Ruth above they welcomed the idea but generally did not find that the homoeopathic practice of Dr Deakin met their needs.

Conversely people who only knew about homoeopathy through the NHS were often not aware of the different model of treatment offered by professional homoeopaths in private practice. So the pluralism of homoeopathy provision tends to be more about chance: coming across it by accident or being recommended by friends; and income, although quite a few of the private homoeopathy users were on relatively low incomes.

The Committed Users appear to be actively seeking a solution from homoeopathy. They had generally ended up in the private sector. When Helen tried to access this different kind of healthcare within the NHS she was disappointed with what was on offer and retreated to the private, non-medical version of homoeopathy. For these users there would be a paradox of attempting to gain access to homoeopathy via the NHS as they are often dissatisfied with biomedicine and are actively seeking an alternative.

Regaining power is one key reason the committed users migrated to private homoeopathy. After disempowering relationships with biomedicine in childbirth, these users reject biomedical technologies, take over more responsibility for healthcare and experience this shift as very empowering. McGuire's (1988) participants in alternative healing systems in suburban America had come to see themselves as 'contractors of their own healthcare' in direct preference over the biomedical passive patient role.

Another reason for seeking homoeopathy outside the NHS is that the philosophy of non-medical homoeopathy seems to be providing some of the users with answers in the search for meaning in their lives and of a missing spiritual dimension. This does not seem to be on offer when a medical GP offers homoeopathy.

In the second group, who appear to be operating a more pragmatic pluralism, there are not the same issues of actively seeking an 'alternative' system. These people are not turning against the authority and power of biomedicine. Far from it, they actually refer to this authority in their use of alternative medicine. They do not appear to be engaged in a search for meaning. Their use of alternative therapies is a purely pragmatic decision where biomedical drugs have not worked or to avoid their side effects, or even in some cases to keep their doctor happy. There is little evidence that their philosophy of health, illness and healing has changed. Their preconceptions are those of the normative biomedical patient with dualistic and mechanistic views of their bodies.

Pluralistic use of medical systems appears to be possible therefore without pluralism of philosophy. Both groups appear to be consistent in their own view of health, healing and the body. Their use of therapies is slotted into this view. Joanne has a very mechanistic view of the body and a very short-term view of treatment. She wants to use homoeopathy 'as a quick fix' for certain symptoms in certain body systems. The committed users and the professional homoeopaths have a different view of their bodies, health and healing. By contrast, for example, they believe that healing may take many years. They come to develop these changed views through their embodied experiences with homoeopathy and their interactions with homoeopaths. I was able to see their views changing particularly clearly in my ethnography of the adult education class.

The only member of the study who has less clearly fixed beliefs about health, healing and the body is Dr Deakin. He appears to be operating both pluralism of practice and philosophy. His multi-level explanations of diagnoses and treatment draw on a number of different philosophies. Perhaps this, along with the lack of time for socialising patients, explains why his patients' views of health, healing and the body remain unchanged. The professional homoeopaths have far more time during their hour long sessions to transmit views of health and healing, to challenge existing beliefs and to educate their patients. This, combined with the fact their patients are often seeking a different way, lead to big changes. The fact that these changes are less obvious in the victim support setting also backs up the importance of time in the consultation. For whilst the half hour appointments here were longer than in general practice, they were still only half the length of private homoeopathic sessions.

Pluralism therefore can be seen both in the health-seeking behaviour and in the offering of healthcare services by providers. Pluralism of use or provision can be associated with a singular health philosophy or with a fragmented plurality of philosophical beliefs. Much of these pluralisms are not commonly understood by users of homoeopathy until they have direct experience.

References

Adams, J. and P. Tovey. 2000. 'Complementary Medicine and Primary Care: Towards a Grassroots Focus', in P. Tovey (ed.) *Contemporary Primary Care: the Challenges of Change*. Buckingham: Open University Press, 167–182.
Amarasingham, L. 1980. 'Movement among Healers in Sri Lanka: a Case Study of Sinhalese Patients', *Culture, Medicine and Psychiatry* 4: 71–92.

Barry, C.A. 2002. 'Identity and Fieldwork: Studying Homoeopathy and Tai Chi "at home" in South London', *Anthropology Matters*, May http://www.anthropologymatters.com/onlinejournal/ChristineBarry.htm.
———2003. 'The Body, Health, and Healing in Alternative and Integrated Medicine: an Ethnography of Homoeopathy in South London'. Unpublished Ph.D. thesis. Brunel University, Uxbridge.
Barry, C.A., C.P. Bradley, N. Britten, F.A. Stevenson and N. Barber. 2000. 'Patients' Unvoiced Agendas in General Practice Consultations: Qualitative Study', *British Medical Journal* 320: 1246–1250.
Barry, C.A., F. Stevenson, N. Britten, N. Barber and C. Bradley. 2001. 'Giving Voice to the Lifeworld. More Humane, More Effective Medical Care?' *Social Science & Medicine* 53: 487–505.
Cant, S. and U. Sharma. 1999. *A New Medical Pluralism? Alternative Medicine, Doctors, Patients and the State*. London: UCL Press.
Castro, M. 1995. *The Complete Homoeopathy Handbook: A Guide to Everyday Health Care*. London: Macmillan.
Dew, K. 2000. 'Deviant Insiders: Medical Acupuncturists in New Zealand', *Social Science & Medicine* 50(12): 1785–1795.
Ernst, E. and A. White. 2000. 'The BBC Survey of Complementary Medicine Use in the UK', *Complementary Therapies in Medicine* 8(1): 32–36.
House of Lords Select Committee on Science and Technology 2000. *Sixth Report: Complementary and Alternative Medicine*. London.
Lindquist, G. 2002. 'Healing Efficacy and the Construction of Charisma: a Family's Journey through the Multiple Medical Fields in Russia', *Anthropology & Medicine* 9(3): 337–358.
McGuire, M.B. 1988. *Ritual Healing in Suburban America*. New Brunswick: Rutgers University Press.
Nicholls, P. 1992. 'Homoeopathy in Britain after the Mid-Nineteenth Century', in M. Saks (ed.) *Alternative Medicine in Britain*. Oxford: Clarendon Press, 77–89.
Porter, R. 1997. *The Greatest Benefit to Mankind: a Medical History of Humanity from Antiquity to the Present*. London: Harper Collins.
Stevenson, F.A., N. Britten, C.A. Barry, C.P. Bradley and N. Barber. 2003. 'Self Treatment and Its Discussion in Medical Consultations: How is Medical Pluralism Managed in Practice', *Social Science & Medicine* 57(3): 513–527.
Thomas, K.J., J.P. Nicholl and M. Fall. 2001. 'Access to Complementary Medicine via General Practice', *British Journal of General Practice* 51: 25–30.
Thomas, K.J., P. Coleman and J.P. Nicholl. 2003. 'Trends in Access to Complementary or Alternative Medicines via Primary Care in England: 1995–2001. Results from a Follow-up National Survey', *Family Practice* 20: 575–577.
Thompson, T.D.B., M.C. Weiss, G. Lewith and D.S. Sharp. 2002. 'Narratives of Engagement. British Medical Doctors Talking about Their Experiences with the Integration of Homoeopathic Medicine into Their Clinical Life'. Paper to 9th Annual Symposium on Complementary Health Care. Dec 4–6, Exeter.
Treuherz, F. 1999. *Homoeopathy in General Practice: a Descriptive Report of Work with 500 Consecutive Patients between 1993–1998*. Northampton: Society of Homoeopaths.
Zollman, C. and A. Vickers. 1999. 'Complementary Medicine in Conventional Practice', *British Medical Journal* 319: 901–904.

7

Re-examining the Medicalisation Process

Efrossyni Delmouzou

My initial interest and preoccupation with the medicalisation legacy and process dates back to my PhD fieldwork[1] in a rural Greek village with the pseudonym of Perachora. Whilst exploring local health-seeking activity I noted that people were unwilling to make their own illness subject of open discussion. Perachorans tended to often medicalise (or demedicalise) their activities claiming and disclaiming being sick according to who was present at the time. At first, I thought that they lacked an appreciation of modern medicine but later it became clear that this was done in hope of preserving their privacy and reputation, which is integral to their survival. In further exploring the people's unwillingness to talk about their health it became clear that they preferred to confine their knowledge to themselves out of fear that others may not hold the same 'medicalisation of ideas' as they did.

It became apparent that the medicalisation process is neither individual nor collective but it is expressed as a function of the individual's relation to the community. This made it extremely difficult for the anthropologist to study the medicalisation process but not impossible. Full-time residents were more prone in hiding illness incidents from the public eye whereas those 'emigrants' who liminally belonged to the village would more readily speak up about their own (or their co-villagers) health problems whilst in Perachora. These 'emigrants' continued to have vested interests in the village but resided for most of the year elsewhere (i.e., Australia, Germany, United States, Athens or Salonica) and did not depend on the local community for work and survival. They readily revealed any information as long as it aided them in their constant struggle of reaffirming their belonging in the village. Thus, they appeared to be well aware of local cultural processes but without realising it, they often breached privacy rules and immensely affected the lives of the full-time residents. As I have argued elsewhere (Delmouzou 1998), full-time residents were equally medicalised in their ideas but were careful of how they talked about their health in public as it impacted on their reputation, their identity, their ability to work and ultimately survive. This chapter builds on these pre-existing arguments and shows that emigrants who reside in Athens full time employ similar tactics to their Perachoran counterparts in keeping illness incidents from the public eye.

Before proceeding let us rehash the medicalisation legacy and process. It is not my aim to evaluate the never-ending literature on medicalisation, which has drawn the attention of many scholars[2] as it would be impossible to do justice properly to all the arguments made on this non-homogeneous process in different times and places within the limitations of a short article. Rather I wish to partly touch on some of the issues that provided the background for 'the medicalisation of ideas'.

Undoubtedly, the availability of medical care and economic circumstances impact on and are indicative of the degree of medicalisation, which is available within a country. In increasingly 'modernising' societies medicalisation is often portrayed as a linear process, deeply dependent and intertwined within the macro level of healthcare (Stacey 1988, Conrad 1992). This to some degree is inherent in the way societies and social organisations function. In societies where the sick role mechanism (see Parsons 1951) is used to control and regulate illness, individuals need to legitimise their withdrawal from the obligations, and to be exempt from any responsibility for their condition. Therefore, in instances where others are unwilling to take the persons own word for the fact that they are ill, medical authorities must intervene in order to validate the claim (Woodward et al. 1995).

In this aforementioned context, scholars began to think of the medicalisation legacy as a linear process that would eventually allow societies to reach the highest possible levels of medicalisation. This trend was often reflected in studies of the effectiveness and efficacy of medicalisation in relation to specific health conditions. The first criticisms of this trend came from Zola and Illich. Zola undoubtedly made the most important contribution, as he was the first scholar to explore the relationship between medical hegemony and the state. He argued that medicalisation was a form of social control, which nudged aside traditional institutions (e.g., religion and law) in the name of health, offering in their place absolute final judgements, which were supposedly morally neutral and objective (Zola 1972: 487). Hence, medicine expands in our private and public lives extending its control over procedures by prescribing drugs and performing surgery, etc. Others like Gerhardt (1989) pointed at its symbolic clinical benefits. Whilst Conrad and Schneider (1980) suggested that the medicalisation of certain conditions may have beneficial characteristics as people may often seek to redefine their problem as an illness to reduce the possible stigma or censure attached to it.

Meanwhile studies of illness which were so to speak in the process achieving their acceptance by the medical community (i.e., chronic fatigue syndrome, etc.) enabled scholars to grasp the medicalisation process as a nonlinear and non-homogenous process which is heavily dependent on the way medical knowledge is constructed. Conrad and Schneider (1980) for instance suggested that the medicalisation process can occur on different levels: at the level of conception when medical language is used; at the institutional level when a problem is legitimised and institutionalised (as a result); and at the consultation level when an actual diagnosis occurs.

> What is less evident however is that conditions warranting health-seeking activity depend on the assessment of the effectiveness of modern medicine, which in turn rests upon implicit definitions of health and illness? This assessment is attempted both by lay people and medical personnel and is often further complicated, when they may be unable to agree with one another (and among themselves) on the cause of the disruption. Incomplete medicalisation may therefore arise when a controversial condition (for instance, chronic fatigue syndrome) arises. (Delmouzou 1998: 16)

The medicalisation process is present both at the individual and the social level. It appears as a component of the global process towards 'modernity'; yet, it is neither homogeneous nor universal. So why is it that in areas with strong medical traditions people do not readily perceive the same 'conditions' as belonging to a specific disease category which is therefore in need of treatment of some kind. Why do people internalise and use medicalisation differently?

It is my contention that the medicalisation process can be better understood if one takes into account the social formations in which 'the medicalisation of ideas' takes place. People working together laying out relations between them can collectively construct knowledge. Likewise, 'the medicalisation of ideas' is also similarly shaped. Hence, it is impossible to look at 'the medicalisation of ideas' without looking at the ways which knowledge is expressed. The interplay between self-knowledge and collective knowledge is important as it impacts on privacy and reputation. Each of us internalises modern medicine differently, according to the circumstances of our lives. We perceive, experience and judge our various actions and ideas in giving meaning to a constructed reality that fits our circumstances and enables our social interactions with others. As I have argued elsewhere:

> 'The medicalisation of ideas' is best seen as a local cultural process. This can be achieved by focusing on how medical ideas are adapted and manifested in expressions and beliefs about health and illness, lying behind value systems and patterns of interpersonal relationships which affect health-seeking activity both at the individual and household level. (Delmouzou 1998: 20)

'The medicalisation of ideas' refers to the acceptance and understanding of medical principles and is a strong indication of whether people view a condition as belonging to specific disease categories that is, therefore, in need of a specifically medical treatment of some kind. Hence, it is evident through the increased use of pharmaceuticals, in the doctor-patient consultations, and in people's willingness to comply with the doctor or seek medical help once, and if, they realise that something is amiss.

'The medicalisation of ideas' also refers to the increased discursive power of biomedicine on the patient's life. 'The medicalisation of ideas' is reflected in health-seeking activities and is mostly evident by the fact that there is a gap between realising that something is amiss and taking action of some kind. People may realise that something is amiss but nonetheless they may rely on his/her own knowledge and experience (e.g., by ignoring the symptoms or using traditional medicine, or using, his/her own medical or biological knowledge). This is only natural, as medicine does not exist in a vacuum. After all, illnesses (and health perceptions) are social and cultural constructs and are interpreted differently according to the sociocultural milieu. Thus, people may often create their own versions of 'medical principles' that are not in agreement with the medical discourse. As in the case that follows, they may rely on their lay medical knowledge.

Scholars tend to study these two perspectives separately but in doing so they fail to see how 'the medicalisation of ideas' affects specific social interrelations existing between the individual, the household and the state. By looking at 'the medicalisation of ideas', we can shed light on the way people engage in health-seeking activities while claiming, and at the same time disclaiming, to be sick depending on whom they talk to. Renewed emphasis can also be given to the selective use of medical ideas and how these are reflected within the household level depending on who is sick and who is judging this. After all the level of distinction between these two perspectives for the lay person depends on multiple factors as is evident in the case study shown below.

The Case of Kimon and Adda

I first met Kimon, an Athenian resident of Kalian descent, in 1994 whilst he was visiting Perachora and over the years we became family friends.[3] A year later, he married Adda from a village in the region of Kalamata. Since their marriage, they continue to reside in Athens but pay long visits to their villages whenever possible. Adda runs a small clothing shop with the help of her mother-in-law and Kimon sells insurance. For the first five years of their marriage, they tried very hard – but unsuccessfully – to have children. This had taken a toll on their relationship and I had suggested on multiple occasions that they should go to an IVF (in vitro fertilization) clinic. Thus far, their lack of action complied with the anthropological literature, which suggests that only a small percentage of health problems reach medical care. People often have to work through their own assumptions and evaluations about their condition (both at the individual level and within their families) before they ask for outside help. At one of their visits they announced whilst adopting quite a medicalised perspective:

Kimon: 'We went to a specialist. He thinks that the problem is twofold on the one hand my sperm is too weak and on the other Adda's ovulation is irregular'. (Athens, February 2000)

Adda: 'I guess this is due to my age as I am now thirty-six years old. Yet the doctor reassured us that with hormone treatment and the new technologies we would soon be pregnant. God knows we've tried everything ranging from alternative medicine to various herbal drinks, foods that are supposed to help. We also made votive offerings[4] to the Virgin Mary in hope that she will grant us a child'. (Athens, February 2000)

From previous informal conversations with the couple I was aware that Adda had tried all viable solutions and her husband had paid the fees incurred without much fuss, as their insurance scheme does not cover nonbiomedical or alternative therapies. In the meantime, she visited at least three gynaecologists and two alternative therapists. She also used multiple types of therapy simultaneously without necessarily worrying about any potential conflicts between the various traditions.[5] Kimon was sure that he would have to cover the cost of this dear therapy on his own. Both had reached a personal understanding and assessment of their condition and were trying to decide on whether to take up treatment with this really expensive doctor who appeared capable of offering promising results. Hence, in my presence they were reassessing their consultation with the doctor.

Kimon: 'We would like your opinion. Does the doctor sound reasonable; do you think there is hope? We have been through so much that I do not want to have false hopes even though my wife reassures me that this man has a reputation of making the impossible possible'. (Athens, February 2000)

I on the other hand felt that this was their decision to make and did not want to influence them in any way:

Efrossyni: 'You must believe in whatever decisions you take in order to achieve the best possible outcome. Just have faith and do not let your anxiety get in the way. I once knew a couple that tried everything in hope of conceiving a child. They finally stopped trying and then a year later she was pregnant. Babies do not always come when we want them but modern medicine can sometimes lend a helping hand.' [Yet even this simple phrase is full of my own 'medical ideas' about the limitations of biomedicine.] (Athens, February 2000)

I was initially introduced to Kimon by his Perachoran grandparents who jokingly stated that they wished to marry him off before they die. From my interviews with them I knew of their intention to leave their house and property directly to their prospective great-grand children so as to make certain that it would remain in the family. They apparently had arranged things so that that the inheritance could not be sold. So I suspected that the couple were under immense pressure. I knew that friends, relatives and other acquaintances often added pressure to the couple by asking questions such as 'when will you decide to have a child?' or less tactfully 'you've been married for some years now and none of you are getting any younger so when will you finally decide to take the next step and become parents?' I also witnessed instances when Kimon and Adda would deflect such questions by suggesting either that they were not ready for the added expenses that children bring with them or by implying that it was not the right time careerwise for them to have kids. In deflecting questions, a legitimate aetiology was used, one that would keep the root of the problem concealed.

Some months later Kimon paid me a visit. I soon found out that he was quite disenchanted with the doctor and felt that the treatment had gone in vain. He asked me to convince Adda to stop the IVF treatment. In his mind, he had already evaluated this therapy as costly and unsuccessful and was no longer willing to comply with the doctor's orders.

This incident points to the ideological and pragmatic considerations that inform therapy choices (Sharma 1992). These may also affect the patient's 'agenda' within the doctor-patient confrontation and have impact on one's willingness to comply with the therapist's orders (Stimson 1974, Stimson and Webb 1975). Patients may for instance try one therapy, evaluate the advantages offered in conjunction with the condition, and then decide if they will continue to use this specific therapy for the health problem. To convince me, Kimon made various compelling revelations about how people present medical incidents and in what context.

Kimon: 'Were you present at our last party [1999] when Adda collapsed from abdominal pain and we had to rush her to the hospital? We told everyone that called to inquire about her health within the next few weeks that she had acute appendicitis. In reality, she actually had an ectopic pregnancy and she was in a bad psychological shape for weeks. If I understood things, correctly, ectopic pregnancies are quite common amongst women and their adverse effects are partly minimised when the problem is detected at an early stage. In Adda's case, however it was too late. ... I think they had to remove her left ovary. That is partly why it has been difficult for us to have children. Do not say anything to my wife about our conversation. She does not want people to know what actually happened even if this explains why we are having difficulties. I keep telling her that she should give up and that we should adopt'. (Athens, July 2000)

Efrossyni: 'She never told me. Your revelation puts Adda's difficulty in a new perspective. Nonetheless, you need not to worry. Adda has done her research and she is well informed about the most beneficial type of treatment. Have faith in the doctor and follow his orders. Adda will not allow herself to be strung along it, she believes she is a hopeless case'. (Athens, July 2000)

Adda kept her ectopic pregnancy from her parents and friends. Her husband firmly believes that she chose to do so because she did not want to be labelled as someone who could not have children of her own. The couple successfully hid the ectopic pregnancy masking it as another illness, which could be resolved through surgery leaving behind no further complications or traces of stigma. The family had enough lay medical knowledge to attribute the distress observed during the party to her appendix. This explanation appeared legitimate to all that were present at the event and the subject was closed. It was also bluntly clear that these people did not lack an appreciation of modern medicine but that their paramount concern was the preservation of their privacy and reputation.

Rather their choice and usage of medical discourse is once again a function of the social relations. Illness narratives might differ in presentation and interpretation depending on the context that they are situated in (Cornwell 1984). This raises a new series of questions for the anthropologists as: 'How "the medicalisation of ideas" is reflected in various narratives?' 'What affects the relationship between lay beliefs and action?'; and 'What is the role of social acceptability in this context?' These cannot be addressed in an article.

Only three people knew that they were trying to conceive with the aid of new reproductive technologies. They would only discuss such sensitive issues in the presence of positive social networks with whom they shared common interests.

A few months later Kimon and Adda took us out for a celebration. Adda was almost two months pregnant and both of them were thrilled. The twins were due in December 2001. Adda made it clear that her pregnancy was to remain a secret for at least another two months as a lot could still go wrong. 'Miscarriages are quite common in the first few moths of pregnancy and we want to know more about the condition of the foetuses before announcing the pregnancy', she said.

During her pregnancy, Adda developed jaundice and the twins were delivered prematurely. Both were around a kilo and had difficulties in breathing so they had to stay in an incubator for more than a month. Nowadays the little girl is almost three. No one would ever guess that she was born prematurely. Unfortunately, however the little boy has a lot of catching up to do. I first noticed the difference in the development of the twins at their Christening. The girl was standing up and sitting but the boy could not sit on his own. Both my husband and I immediately felt something was amiss. The comparison between our child, who was also born prematurely, and the two twins was shocking. This same nagging feeling was present every time we saw the twins but any talk about the development of the boy was deflected. Adda kept stressing how pleased she was with the twins' development and how the neonatal team had congratulated them on the progress.

Six months later only the little girl came to my son's party whereas her twin brother who had the flue stayed at home so as not to spread any germs around. This seemed a legitimate excuse at the time on behalf of the mother. The first indication that the couple was aware that something was amiss came on another occasion. Kimon openly complained about the development of his son.

Kimon: 'I do not know what is going to happen with this boy. He took longer than his sister did to sit up and he had to undergo physiotherapy as his limbs were too stiff and he is only now gradually attempting to walk on his own. We thought that we had put this problem behind us. What worries me is that the doctors are not pleased with how he reacts to his surrounding. He plays with his sister quite a bit, but she is a better communicator than he is. He seems to envy things she does that he cannot. Sometimes he tries to replicate her actions but most of the time he chooses to tune out and hide in his own little world. Adda decided to take the kids to her parents' house for a month. The house is a bit secluded from the rest of the town but the clean air and the sea will do these kids a great deal of good. Besides our boy will get extra attention from his grandparents and cousins. As for me, I visit my children on weekends. The doctors have urged us to spend more time playing with our son, to further his development. Unfortunately, I cannot afford a vacation even though I really missed Kalis in the six years that have lapsed from my last visit... Hopefully I will be able to visit Kalis next year; by then the children will be almost three and easier to handle. They will be older and hopefully my son's poor development will be less noticeable'. (Athens, August 2003)

Efrossyni: 'I can see that you are concerted about public reaction but I think it is unfair to expect premature babies to show the development of children who have reached full term at birth. You have done a wonderful job so far. No one will ever guess that the girl was born prematurely, she walks steadily and she speaks very clearly for her age. Besides boys do not develop at the same rate as girls do....'

He interrupted me before I could continue the sentence.

Kimon: 'Yes but the comparison between them is devastating and people will surely notice the difference and they may attribute it to hereditary issues. We have already attracted village gossip because we were married for more than five years before we decided to have any children, so I do not want them questioning our involvement with them'. (Athens, August 2003)

I was once again in the process of suggesting that they should get another medical opinion when Kimon abruptly changed the topic of the conversation as my husband entered the house. This is only natural as the two men were not familiar with one another. I was left with an uncomfortable impression, which grew stronger as I recalled that Kimon's home was nearby the village square where children play. Kimon was trying to hide his family's health problem. It was obvious that he did not want to attract the attention of others who do not necessarily share the same 'medicalisation of ideas' as they did. Most probably the couple had chosen a wait-and-see tactic concerning their son.

My husband politely enquired about his family. Kimon typically replied that they were all fine. The two men exchanged a few more words about cars and insurances. Upon leaving Kimon stated: 'The twins have grown a lot; on my next visit I will bring them over so that they can play with your son'.

His words hit me like a block. I suddenly felt as if I was in Perachora, a remote village were people would either claim or disclaim their sickness according to who is present at the time. Alternatively, they confined their knowledge to themselves out of fear that the villagers may not necessarily hold the same 'medicalisation of ideas' as they did. Perachorans preferred to discuss things with those who held the same 'medicalisation of ideas' as they did.

Once again, privacy plays a central role with regards to ill health. In the presence of others, people's medicalised ideas may be temporarily altered for the purpose of concealment and protection. People may more readily share and express their ideas with others, (which to them) seem to display the same level of 'medicalisation of ideas', especially those that appear to have an understanding of medical knowledge (and an evaluation of it) which resembles their own understanding or evaluation. Reputation construction can also be contingent to these strategies.

Looking at the medicalisation process through a different prism

Throughout the aforementioned case study, we have seen how 'the medicalisation of ideas' impacts on the couple's decisions about whether or not they need to engage in health seeking activities. It affects decisions about the most appropriate treatment and forms an evaluative basis. The impact of 'the medicalisation of ideas' is also evident in the interpretations of the nature and cause of illness, its severity and type (Lasker 1981, Sharma 1992) and the evaluation of the best possible cure. 'The medicalisation of ideas' is also related to pragmatic considerations (e.g., cost, accessibility) as these inform decisions about health (ibid.).

Moreover, 'the medicalisation of ideas' is also constrained by considerations of privacy. Issues of illness are often covered with reserve, as they are dependent on shared notions of morality. Hence even though people seldom take health decisions by themselves (Sharma 1992) extra care may be taken in 'lay referral' (Freidson 1961).

Kimon's and Adda's case is by no means unique. Perachoran and Kalian decendents residing in Athens often displayed similar health-seeking activities as their village counterparts. People displayed various medical ideas at various times. These were shaped and reshaped according to the situation. Moreover, claiming and disclaiming being sick appeared as a function of the person's social relations. If a great deal of privacy is perceived as needed they may turn to the most readily available method (e.g., treating the complaint at home) even if it is less effective.

In such cases 'lay referral' (Freidson 1961) is limited to the immediate family and particularly to those who share similar ideas about medicalisation. Moreover, outside help is used in severe, chronic cases (Lasker 1981) or when a patient fails to recover; but those involved are carefully selected.

Within the wider urban setting of Athens, positive and negative relationships were harder to spot and the impact of the health-seeking activities was not always as visible as in the village or in other more bounded settings. Fieldwork in such settings requires that a good rapport is reached between the informant, the researcher, and his wider circle of acquaintances, which will span for several years. Despite these difficulties, similar findings were often reaffirmed. Once again, even in urban settings 'the medicalisation of ideas' is not independent from privacy and reputation. This observation enabled me to make some assumptions from the point of view of the individual agent regardless of his relation to the community.

First, that many societies nowadays display some degree of medical pluralism and permit some sort of access to modern medicine, or to alternative and traditional healing solutions. Second, we need to remember that people depend on their beliefs and experiences when they intentionally and unintentionally medicalise their condition. Increasingly lay people in 'modern' societies have the ability to inform themselves about beneficial types of treatments and their appropriateness (Lock 1980) when they realise that they are in need of professional care or that something is amiss. Third, 'the medicalisation of ideas' requires some sort of internalisation, acculturation and adoption of some medical concepts (which may not necessarily be in agreement with official medical knowledge) amongst lay people. When they are either maintaining and/or ameliorating their health these people should be willing to utilise these concepts (on their own or together with other traditional healing systems). Fourth, we do not need to assume that a high level of 'medicalisation of ideas' will necessarily bring people running to hospitals or medical practitioners, for, as it is suggested in the anthropological literature, people have their own assumptions and evaluations of their condition. Moreover, only a small percentage of health problems reach medical care. Fifth, visiting the doctor (or other medical personnel) for therapeutic purposes or for advice does not result in automatic compliance with the doctor's orders. Lay people will turn to their own medicalised ideas in order to evaluate such consultations (perhaps more than once and with the aid of others). Compliance and non-compliance heavily depend on such evaluations, which may also entail a reshaping of the pre-existing medicalised ideas. Sixth, medicalised ideas are not static nor do they exist in a vacuum. They are created, changed and reshaped by our interactions with other lay people and with medical personnel.

In this process, the contribution of science and the mass media cannot be ignored but medicalisation is not a collective process. We must not forget that health-seeking activity and sickness/illness prevention are experienced from a number of vantage points as well as within social and cultural constraints. As I have argued elsewhere,[6] our medicalised ideas entail attempt(s) to construct a worldview in an acceptable manner, whilst simultaneously reflecting how we see the world, and how we judge others in their transformations of bodily suffering or health maintenance (Delmouzou 1998: 27).

Each individual agent upholds his/her own 'medicalisation of ideas' depending on the health related incidents that they face. Nevertheless, the implications of this health-seeking activity are neither individual nor collective. Rather they are expressed as a function of the individual's relation to the community. This realisation raises extra demands for the anthropologist. In the past, medical anthropologists were predominantly concerned with the collective structure of health, with an emphasis on identifying common ideas about health and illness (Blum and Blum 1965, Helman 1986, Janzen 1978, Lewis 1975, Ohnuki-Tierney 1984). Recently we appear to be preoccupied with individual people and narratives (for instance, studies concerned with the individual assimilation of ideas and consumer satisfaction reports) (Brown 1992, Calnan et al. 1994). Yet, it seems to me that in doing so we have forgotten that emphasis should be placed on how individual and community affect one another.

In Kimon's and Adda's case, and in many others like it, 'the medicalisation of ideas' is expressed in the interactions of the individual's relation to the community. These interactions impact on how knowledge is embedded in local medical ideas, and how it is adopted and displayed according to context or according to who is present.

Notes

1. Which was conducted 1994–1998.
2. for example, Arney and Bergen 1984, Bell 1990, Binney et al. 1990, Britten 1995, Broom and Woodward 1996, Conrad 1992, Conrad and Schneider 1980, Crawford 1980, Freidson 1986, Illich 1990, Lowenberg and Davis 1994, Oinas 1998, Rieff 1987, Szasz 1970, Zola 1972.
3. It is through this friendship that I became privy to their experiences and convinced Kimon and Adda to allow me to use their example as a case study. To convince them I argued that it is linked to my previous work as it reveals how Perachorans' descendents often use the same tactics as their village counterparts. Further examples and information on the social context of Perachorans can be found in my PhD thesis and forthcoming book. However, I cannot reveal anymore specific information about this couple without violating the very privacy that they were seeking to maintain. This article is based on informal interviews and note taking but also depends on other observations and knowledge facilitated by previous fieldwork.
4. Believers often ask the various Saints or the Virgin Mary to grant them a miracle that will improve their health or wellbeing. If an infant is saved or born they may name it after the Saint or they may in return give other votive offering to the divinity that came to their aid (see also Dubish 1995).
5. Similar observations were made by Amarasingham-Rhodes 1980.
6. In my PhD thesis (Delmouzou 1998) and forthcoming book (Delmouzou Forthcoming).

References

Amarasingham-Rhodes, L. 1980. 'Movement among Healers in Sri Lanka: a Case Study of a Sinhalese Patient', *Culture Medicine & Psychiatry* 4: 71–9.
Arney, W.R. and B.J. Bergen. 1984. *Medicine and the Management of Living.* Chicago: University of Chicago Press.

Bell, S.E. 1990. 'Sociological Perspectives on the Medicalisation of Menopause', *Annals New York Academy of Sciences* 592: 173–78.

Binney, E.A., C.L. Estes and S.R. Ingman. 1990. 'Medicalisation, Public Policy and the Elderly: Social Science in Jeopardy?' *Social Science & Medicine* 30: 761–771.

Blum, H.R. and M.E. Blum. 1965. *Health and Healing in Rural Greece.* Stanford: Stanford University Press.

Britten, N. 1995. 'Lay Views of Drugs and Medicines: Orthodox and Unorthodox Accounts', in S.J. Williams and M. Calnan (eds) *Modern Medicine: Lay Perspectives and Experiences.* London: UCL Press, 48–73.

Broom, H.D. and V.R. Woodward. 1996. 'Medicalisation Reconsidered: Towards a Collaborative Approach to Health Care', *Sociology of Health And Illness* 18(3): 357–378.

Brown, P.E. 1992. 'Symptoms and Social Performances: The Case of Diane Reden', in M.D. Good, P.E. Brodwin, B.J. Good and A. Kleinman (eds) *Pain as Human Experience: An Anthropological Perspective.* Berkeley: Berkley University of California Press, 77–99.

Calnan, M., V. Katsouyiannopoulos, V.K. Ovcharov, R. Prokhorshas, H. Ramic and S. Williams. 1994. 'Major Determinants of Consumer Satisfaction with Primary Health Care in Different Health Systems', *Family Practice* 11(4): 468–478.

Conrad, P. 1992. 'Medicalisation and Social Control', *Annual Review of Sociology* 18: 209–232.

Conrad, P. and J.W Schneider. 1980. *Deviance and Medicalisation: From Badness to Sickness.* St. Louis: CV Mosby.

Cornwell, J. 1984. *Hard-earned Lives.* London: Tavistock.

Crawford, R. 1980. 'Healthism and the Medicalisation of Everyday Life', *International Journal of Health Care Services* 10(3): 365–388.

Delmouzou, E. 1998. 'An Ethnographic Approach to Health-Seeking Activity in Rural Greece.' Unpublished Ph.D. thesis. University of Derby, U.K.

Delmouzou, E. (Forthcoming) 'Morgaged Lives and Reputations: Privacy, Health and Identity'.

Dubisch, J. 1995. *In a Different Place: Pilgrimage, Gender and Politics of A Greek Island Shrine.* Princeton: Princeton University Press.

Freidson, E. 1961. *Patient Views of Medical Practice. A Study of Subscribers to a Prepaid Medical Plan in the Bronx.* New York: Russell Sage Foundation.

Freidson, E. 1986. 'The Medical Profession in Transition.', in L.H. Aiken and D. Mechanic (eds) *Applications of Social Science to Clinical Medicine and Health Policy.* New Brunswick, New Jersey: Rutgers University Press, 63–79.

Gerhardt, U. 1989. 'The Sociological Image of Medicine and the Patient', *Social Science & Medicine* 29(6): 721–728.

Helman, C. 1986. ' "Feed a Cold, Starve a Fever": Folk Models of Infection in an English Suburban Community, and their Relations to Medical Treatment', in C. Currer and M. Stacey (eds) *Concepts of Health, Illness and Disease.* Oxford: Oxford Berg, 213–231.

Illich, I. 1990. *Limits to Medicine: Medical Nemesis: The Exploration of Health and Death.* London: Penguin Books.

Janzen, J.M. 1978. *The Quest of Therapy in Lower Zaire.* Berkeley: University of California Press.

Lasker, J. (1981) 'Choosing among Therapies: Illness Behaviour in the Ivory Coast', *Social Science & Medicine*, 15A: 157–168.

Lewis, G. 1975. *Knowledge of Illness in a Sepik Society.* London: The Athlone Press.

Lock, M. 1980. *East Asian Medicine in Urban Japan.* Berkeley: University of California Press.

Lowenberg, S.J. and F. Davis. 1994. 'Beyond Medicalisation-demedicalisation. The Case of Holistic Health', *Sociology of Health And Illness* 16(5): 579–599.

Ohnuki-Tierney, E. 1984. *Illness and Culture in Contemporary Japan: An Anthropological View.* Cambridge: Cambridge University Press.

Oinas, E. 1998. 'Medicalisation by Whom? Accounts of Menstruation Conveyed by Young Women and Medical Experts in Medical Advisory Columns', *Sociology of Health and Illness* 20(1): 52–70.

Parsons, T. 1951. *The Social System.* New York: Free Press.

Rieff, P. 1987. *The Triumph of the Therapeutic: Uses of Faith After Freud.* Chicago: University of Chicago Press.

Sharma, U. 1992. *Complementary Medicine Today: Practitioners and Patients.* London: Routledge.

Stacey, M. 1988. *The Sociology of Health and Healing.* London: Unwin.

Stimson, V.G. 1974. 'Obeying Doctor's Orders: A View form the Other Side', *Social Science & Medicine* 8: 94–104.

Stimson, V.G. and B. Webb. 1975. *Going to See the Doctor.* London: Routledge & Kegan Paul.

Szasz, T.S. 1970. *The Manufacture of Madness.* New York: Harper.

Woodward, R., H.D. Broom and D.G. Leggee. 1995. 'Diagnosis in Chronic Illness: Disabling or Enabling – The Case of Chronic Fatigue Syndrome', *Journal of the Royal Society of Medicine* 88(179/94a): 1–6.

Zola, K.I. 1972. 'Medicine as an Institution of Social Control', *Sociological Review* 20: 487–503.

Part II

Body, Self and the
Experience of Healing

8

Healing and the Mind-body Complex
Childbirth and Medical Pluralism in South Asia

Geoffrey Samuel

This article attempts to put together two bodies of work I did at different times. The first was a kind of rethinking of anthropological theorising about mind, body and culture which was undertaken originally in the late 1980s in the context of a study of religion in Tibetan societies (Samuel 1990a, 1990b).

The second area of research was in medical anthropology. In the late 1990s I undertook some research on medical pluralism in a Tibetan refugee community in North India (Samuel 1999, 2001a), and subsequently edited a book on childbirth in South and Southeast Asia along with my partner, Santi Rozario (Rozario and Samuel 2002a). I shall refer to some of the South and Southeast Asian childbirth research below.

Medical anthropology has had a complex ongoing relationship with the Western medical tradition (henceforward referred to as biomedicine). This is often a one-sided relationship and not always a comfortable one. On the one side, medical anthropologists see themselves as having a wider and more inclusive context within which to place healing practices of all kinds, including those of biomedicine. Medical anthropologists feel that biomedical practice is often severely weakened in its effectiveness by a lack of awareness of this wider context. On the other side, biomedical practitioners tend to see biomedicine as a relatively self-contained and scientifically validated body of procedures, to which medical anthropology is a marginal add-on. I am exaggerating a little here, since there is certainly more dialogue today than a few years ago. There is still plenty of truth in my description, however, even in the more progressive Western medical contexts, let alone in many South Asian situations. Even where medical anthropology is accepted, it is more for its knowledge of the social context of biomedicine than for its ability to relativise and critique biomedical procedures through anthropological analysis.

Some of this, of course, is straightforward politics, both politics within universities, and the larger politics of access to development funding. What I concentrate on here, though, is rather different. This is the way in which the biomedical perspective is unable, because of its own internal logic, to admit an understanding of the cultural level as other than a marginal addition. I suggest that this inability arises because biomedical explanation is essentially posed at the level of the body. Mental and emotional factors are by definition secondary within a perspective whose central focus is on the maintenance of the homoeostatic processes of *bodily* functioning.

This means that modes of healing that do not fit easily into this body-centred framework (I am thinking particularly of healing practices based on ideas such as spirit-agency or soul-loss) make no sense. Neither do the characteristic modes of analysis of cultural and social anthropology, which equally give mental, emotional or cultural factors primacy. That 'mind' may affect 'body' to some degree can scarcely be denied, but as long as 'mind' and 'body' are regarded as separate entities, and the basic paradigm of explanation is at the level of the body – of physiology – then any critique is blunted and defused. Cultural analysis, by contrast, tends to deal pre-eminently with the mental and emotional.

Thus biomedicine can manage a limited dialogue with the classic humoral-medical systems of Asia – Galenic-Islamic, Ayurvedic, Tibetan and Chinese – because, in effect, they work on much the same terms as itself, if within a somewhat expanded view of relevant factors and interconnections. When, however, we turn from these sophisticated and literate humoral systems to look at the area of spirit causation and spiritual agency more generally, we have moved into a different framework of analysis, and one that it is hard to see as compatible with conventional biomedicine. Typically, the biomedical reaction to spirit causation, soul-loss or similar conceptions of illness causation is to regard the theory as nonsense, and any therapeutic effect as part of the famous and mostly unanalysed 'placebo effect'. Patients improve because they believe that they have been treated with an effective remedy. We have no idea why this happens in general, why it may happen in some cases but not in others, or what specifically there might have been about the treatment that might have been conducive to a positive outcome.

Ironically, this is one of the areas where anthropology has most to say, which makes the lack of communication between biomedicine and anthropology at this point the more regrettable. Much anthropological work on spirit causation focuses on what we might term psychological illness (e.g., Kapferer 1979, 1983) but in fact spirit-related treatment modalities are by no means restricted to psychological complaints.

While working towards an analysis of religion in Tibetan societies some years ago, I developed a framework of analysis that began from the opposite assumption to biomedicine: that any explanation had to be phrased in terms of mind, body, social and physical environment *as a whole*; that the separation between mind and body, and for that matter between self and other, had to be taken as both secondary and as specific to particular individuals and cultural contexts. This was because I saw the ritual procedures of Tibetan Buddhism as acting upon this mind-body-society-environment complex as a whole, on what might be called in Gregory Bateson's phrase 'the ecology of mind' (Bateson 1973). In this, I suggested, they were typical of a whole class of procedures, which could be called 'shamanic' for want of a better term, which operated in this way.

Obviously, such a framework cuts across our existing vocabulary, particularly in English and most European languages, and so it involved me in developing an alternative vocabulary of analytic concepts. The results were presented in a book (Samuel 1990a); there is also a short account on my website (Samuel 1990b). The key feature was a vocabulary of *states* of the mind-body-society-environment complex. These states (I called them *modal states*) could be seen both as *cultural* states (for example, one might think of the typical 'states,' physical, mental, emotional, of a South Asian extended family in rural Bangladesh), but could also be seen as a repertoire of *personal* states possessed by each individual, and learned and internalised during their lifetime.

The very nature of the 'individual', however, is itself a function of these states, since they define for the individual how individuality and subjectivity are experienced, and how the mind-body complex functions in relation to the wider social group and physical environment. Being, for example, a young wife in an extended family household in North India or Bangladesh is defined by a whole series of patterned relationships with other members of the household as well as with non-members (see, for example, Jeffery and Jeffery 1993 for Uttar Pradesh, North India; Kotalová 1993 for Bangladesh; Lamb 2000: 42–69 for West Bengal). The young wife has specific relations of deference, service and compliance towards her husband, her mother-in-law, father-in-law, and other kinds of patterned relationships with her husband's elder brother and his wife, her husband's younger siblings and their spouses if any, and so on. Equally, she has expectations of specific forms of behaviour in response from each of these persons.

These relationships are learned or acquired through the individual's personal life experience. They allow a certain scope – often quite limited, as in this case – for the individual to express or assert herself. Yet – and I think these are important points – each individual learns how to negotiate these patterned relationships in a slightly different way. This is the basis perhaps of what we experience as 'personality'.

In a contemporary middle-class Western European household, the expectations may be less conscious and formalised, and the scope for individual expression somewhat wider, though the cultural models provided by family, television or advertising still play a very strong part (Samuel 1990a: 140–141). All of these ways can, at least in principle, change as long as the individual is alive.

This is a language that is well adapted to talk about spirit healing and similar processes, since it was designed in part to make better sense of anthropological theorising in this area.

Elsewhere (Samuel 2001b) I have discussed one particular anthropological tradition – the analysis of spirit-healing, which derives initially from studies such as Claude Lévi-Strauss' 1949 paper 'The Effectiveness of Symbols' (Lévi-Strauss 1977) and Turner's work on African ritual (e.g., Turner 1968, 1969, 1970) – and suggested how this tradition can be reformulated and made more coherent in terms of a framework of modal states. Here I will simply take this reformulation for granted, except to point out that cultural 'symbols' (including spirits) can be seen as referencing, and so enabling a healer to operate on and with, the states of which I am speaking. To put this in other words, spirits can be seen as labels for kinds of relationships with one's own mind-body complex, with other people and with other aspects of one's environment. Culturally specified modes of interaction with spirits (possession and exorcism, spirit-mediumship, shamanic encounters, etc.) can thus provide ways of transforming and renegotiating these relationships. Such renegotiating may be an essential part of a healing process.

Childbirth in South Asia

Lévi-Strauss' analysis in 'The Effectiveness of Symbols' was specifically to do with a shamanic ritual for a difficult childbirth. While there are certainly problems with his analysis, as subsequent authors have noted, I think that there is an important point here which I have tried to take up and reformulate (Samuel 2001b). The point is that the cultural material presented to the birthing mother, whether specifically in the context of a healing intervention, or more generally in the way her culture and the people around her manage childbirth, will have an effect on her ability to deal herself with the process of childbirth.

I move now specifically to the South Asian material on childbirth. This is a difficult and contested area of study, particularly in regard to rural areas where most children continue to be born at home with the assistance of a traditional birth attendant (called *dai* in many parts of North India and Bangladesh). In fact, as most authorities are well aware, the high rates of mortality and morbidity among both mothers and children in the region have more to do with poor diet and the lack of basic public health measures such as clean water and adequate sanitation than with the unavailability of high-technology biomedical interventions (Samuel 2002: 17, 29 n.19).

Any assessment of the relative value of traditional childbirth practices and biomedicine is nevertheless a complex business. The 'traditional' practices – at least as we encounter them today – involve negative and problematic features, especially in North India and Bangladesh. Many of these derive from the strong linkage between childbirth and pollution, and the associated attitude towards traditional birth attendants. Thus in Patricia Jeffery, Roger Jeffery and Andrew Lyon's well-known North Indian study 'Labour Pains and Labour Power' (1989) we read that the *dai* 'does not have overriding control over the management of deliveries. Nor is she a sisterly and supportive equal. Rather she is a low status menial necessary for removing defilement' (Jeffery et al. 1989: 108). As has since been emphasised, this description is a representation of local views and in no sense the authors' own judgment of the village *dais* and their skills (Jeffery et al. 2002: 93). In reality, many *dais* undoubtedly acquire real expertise, either from training or experience.

Janet Chawla has argued persuasively against taking this language of pollution at face value. Thus the time between birth and the ritual that ends post-birth pollution (called *chhati* in Bihar and much of North India) is called *narak ka samay* by the *dais*. Literally, this means the time of *narak*. *Narak* is the normal word for hell or underworld, but Chawla suggests that it can be seen in this context as the 'site/energy of the unseen inner world' and that it 'signifies the fertility or fruitful potential of the earth and the female body' (Chawla 2002: 159–160). Similarly, terms such as *gandagi* ('filth') are part of a diagnostic vocabulary for the *dai* and do not have the negative meanings they would have for the Brahmanic tradition.

Chawla's point is well taken. The Brahmanic tradition is only one of many discourses within Indian society, and it is important to avoid the temptation to read Indian culture exclusively through it. The Brahmanic language of purity and pollution is nevertheless closely associated with the status hierarchy of South Asian societies, Muslim as well as Hindu, and it seems clear that traditional birth attendants are routinely disparaged and devalued because of their linkage with the polluting business of childbirth.

Thus Rozario describes the low status of traditional birth attendants in Bangladesh and the ways in which they attempt to counter these in their own lives (Rozario 2002). The counterpart of this low status is that young, educated women are unlikely to take on these roles, and that the older, uneducated women who do act as birth attendants, whatever their actual level of expertise, may have limited ability to insist on their advice being followed.[1]

If 'traditional' birthing practices in South Asia can be problematic, so often is the provision of biomedicine, where it is available at all. Difficulties here relate both to what is provided and the context in which it is provided. Village-level medical practitioners may have limited training and their intervention may be restricted to providing oxytocin injections and the like without physically examining the woman in any way. Hospitals are frequently unhygienic, dangerous and expensive, and the attitudes of their largely urban medical staff to rural women can be dismissive and unsympathetic, as well as disrespectful of local norms of propriety and behaviour. Since urban doctors and nurses are, like the village 'doctors', unwilling to come into direct contact with women's bodies, hospital births may in fact be assisted by untrained *ayahs* without any medically trained personnel being present (Afsana and Rashid 2000: 35, 65–66, 102). These features have been documented by a wide range of studies (e.g., Rozario 1995, Afsana and Rashid 2000, see also Samuel 2002).

The situation in relation to both traditional and biomedical practices appears to be rather better in South India. Here 'traditional' practices seem less dominated by pollution concerns and negative attitudes towards female bodily functions, and hospital provision is also often better, though there is still an ongoing tension between the discourses of modernity and local cultural practices surrounding childbirth (Ram 2001, van Hollen 2002, 2003).

Mind-body states in childbirth

I have been struck, however, by the extent to which the various researchers in this area seem to find themselves caught up within the incompatibility of biomedical and cultural frameworks that I sketched in the opening sections of this paper (see, for example, Chawla 1994, 2002, Jeffery et al. 1989, Jeffery et al. 2002, Unnithan-Kumar 1999, 2002). Could the framework I have outlined be of any help in giving a clearer view of the overall situation? Such an approach would involve looking at childbirth practices in South Asia simultaneously in terms of physiology, and in terms of what these practices communicate to the birthing mother and other participants in the childbirth about how to make sense of the process of childbirth.

I mention other participants deliberately, since the behaviour of other family members in particular may be a critical part of the situation. A birthing woman in a South Asian extended family is rarely in a position to make decisions by herself, particularly if she is young, and least of all once childbirth is already in progress. However, for simplicity I will concentrate here on the birthing mother herself.

A woman's body goes through dramatic physical and hormonal changes during birth, which the woman has to make sense of, understand and deal with (and here I am particularly thinking about her first birth). In other words, she has to create a rational and emotional understanding of what is going on at the physical level – a series of modal states, in terms of the framework I sketched earlier.

So the question becomes, 'what is the material from which she is going to construct those modal states and that understanding?' The body does not feel in abstract terms. We are always making sense of what is going on through images, giving cognitive and emotional meaning to our hormonal and physical states. While hormonal changes and other physiological processes are closely linked to emotion, they are not the same thing. Patterns of hormonal flow and other physiological processes strongly shape the 'modal states', but they do not determine them, and this is where the 'cultural' factors enter, both the way in which the childbirth itself is handled (cf. Lévi-Strauss 1977, Laderman 1987), and the wider set of ideas surrounding childbirth and other female bodily processes.

Thus, for example, the 'states' developed by the woman encompass her interaction with the people around her and so are developed in interaction with those other people and their own established ways of behaving, thinking and feeling. These are in turn linked to general cultural ideas and practices concerning the meaning of childbirth. Thus ideas about childbirth being a normal process, and about the need for women to deal with labour pains silently and without making any fuss, are widespread in South Asia and can be found throughout the ethnographic accounts:

> What [will] other people [...] think if one shouts like an uncivilised person? What do you expect from them if you do not behave yourself? Even the *dhaitani* [traditional birth attendant] gets annoyed and scolds the woman bitterly, if she is not properly behaved. To be well mannered women should tolerate their pain (Afsana and Rashid 2000: 55, comment by a rural woman in Bangladesh).

> The common image of a labouring woman in Mogra is one who endures her agony silently. The not-yet-mothers appropriate this image much earlier in life. Young girls witness child deliveries and overhear adult women discussing pregnancies and child deliveries occurring in their neighbourhood. A woman facing prolonged labour pain knows what is expected of her and of those attending on her... Child delivery is handled with a matter-of-course attitude, and this indeed is the cultural ideal (Patel 1994: 110, on Rajasthan).

Tulsi Patel also notes that any complications with the birth are thought to imply that the woman's behaviour has been at fault.

> The belief is so deeply internalised that labouring women consciously suppress their anguish to avoid being labelled as bad. They set an example of courage and fortitude. Even summoning any outside help is avoided as long as possible. Calling a *dai* is considered the first signal of difficulty, while calling a nurse is a strong indication that the woman is not noble. After a few childbirths many women prefer to deliver their babies without a *dai*'s or nurses help, to demonstrate that child delivery is not difficult (Patel 1994: 120).

At the same time, Patel stresses the warm and supportive environment provided by family members, which she regards as reducing the birthing woman's anxiety and fear.

If, as Patel suggests, concepts regarding childbirth are acquired at an early age through witnessing births and listening to adult women talking about them, they are also signalled by the specific practices associated with birth. These include rituals such as the *cimantam* ritual performed in Tamil Nadu in preparation for a woman's first birth (van Hollen 2003: 76–79), and the various rituals and behaviours that may be performed in order to assist a difficult birth. They also include the dietary and other practices linked with the widespread South and Southeast Asian idea that the transition of childbirth is associated with a transition of the woman's body from 'hot' to 'cold' in humoral terms.

This transition is marked in diet and in other respects. While cold here strictly speaking does not refer literally to temperature but to a quality within the humoral system, it is often associated, particularly in Southeast Asia, with an emphasis on keeping the mother warm in the period after birth or even subjecting her to considerable heat by keeping her close to a fire, the so-called 'mother-roasting' practices discussed by Manderson and others (Manderson 1981).

In South Asia, it is more generally a question of taking 'cooling' foods and avoiding 'heating' foods during pregnancy, since 'overheating' the woman might interfere with the pregnancy or injure the child (e.g., Hutter 1994: 151–153), and adopting the opposite regime after birth – though it has to be added that in the impoverished conditions of many South Asian households, all this may be more an ideal than a reality (cf. Unnithan-Kumar 2002). Special foods are supplied, such as the sweet *laddu* compounded of a variety of herbal and other ingredients given to the birthing mother in Rajasthan and elsewhere.

Women today vary in their attitudes to these food restrictions and prescriptions. They clearly often find them irksome and see no need to follow them if they can avoid having to:

> In the interview with K. she said she does eat banana, etcetera during pregnancy. We asked whether she, like other women, believed that it would lead to illness of the child or not. She said she just eats everything and does not bother. At that moment, an elderly lady (family member) came in and listened to us. Then, K. suddenly starts to use sentences like 'one should not take banana' and 'they say one should not take…' In this way, K. paid respect to the elderly lady, and pretended that she avoided these food items during pregnancy although in reality she did not (Hutter 1994: 161).

Women after birth may have less choice over their diet: Maya Unnithan-Kumar notes that in the community she studied in Rajasthan, 'a new mother (*jaccha*) is prohibited from touching the hearth and water pots due to pollution arising from childbirth which can be active for up to forty days. She is thus dependent on other women feeding her' (Unnithan-Kumar 2002: 121). Unnithan-Kumar also notes that:

> Mothers, mothers-in-law and elder sisters-in-law give advice on which and what quantities of special foods are to be eaten in the eighth month of pregnancy. These include, for example, coconut, sesame seed oil and castor oil because of their lubricating properties which would help the foetus move easily within the womb to ensure a smooth delivery. Only women who are grandmothers or who have pregnant daughters are aware of the ingredients of the special sweetmeat (*ladoo*), compulsory for women to ingest after the birth. Jetoon told me her mother put thirty-two different items in it but could name only a few. Kamlesh said normally thirty to forty of such sweetmeat balls are made, one for every day after the birth until normal food was resumed. Jetoon said she never ate hers because she did not like the taste, so in fact they were all eaten by her children instead (ibid: 121).

What is important to appreciate is that we can understand what is going on here at two different levels, though they cannot in fact be entirely separated from each other. At one level, the changes in diet, external temperature, and the like, have an actual physiological effect (assuming that the dietary rules are actually obeyed, which clearly varies). How substantial this effect might be, and how far it might be in directions that make sense in biomedical terms, is difficult to say. Some authors have argued that the food restrictions after childbirth, in Bangladesh and North India at any rate, are likely to have a harmful effect, if only in that they prevent the mother from taking more nutritious items in the local diet. Unnithan-Kumar's chapter on Rajasthan portrays a situation where almost all women are chronically undernourished, and are in fact further under cultural pressure to reduce their diet because of ideas that overeating may have a bad effect on their breast milk (Unnithan-Kumar 2002). Van Hollen's description of Tamil Nadu, a region where the general level of nutrition is probably considerably better than in Rajasthan to begin with, suggests that, at the least, some biomedical opinions of the harmfulness of post-partum dietary restrictions are unfounded. I see no reason to assume that the folk medical and Ayurvedic dietary prescriptions and restrictions, in Tamil Nadu at any rate, are not having some positive effect – as van Hollen notes, these rules are applied in a flexible way and are open to experimentation and experience (van Hollen 2002).

Leaving this level of the physiological effect of dietary practices aside, there is also a second level, in which the dietary practices have a symbolic meaning, where they are communicating something to the mother and to those who are looking after her. As her body undergoes the major change from advanced pregnancy to the post-partum state and the commencement of breastfeeding, the changes in diet, along with associated ritual practices, such as the *Shasthi* or *Bemata* rituals that take place six days or so after childbirth and mark the end of childbirth pollution (Rozario and Samuel 2002b: 187–190, see also Hutter 1994: 185–187), are also signalling these major changes to the mother and her carers. Table 8.1 provides a general picture of how these various phases, activities and concepts relate to each other. The two major transitional phases (birth and the end of confinement) are marked in grey.

As I said, one cannot entirely separate these two levels: the physiological effect of the food, for example, may well be affected by how the food is received emotionally – as a message of care and concern, perhaps. Both together build up the modal state, or rather provide the mother with 'material' from which she will build up the state (in a largely unconscious manner, as with all modal-state production). Women understand their experiences in terms of this material. Thus a mother in Karnataka speaks in relation to her birth of how 'all the heat has gone during delivery. I lost a lot of blood so there is no *kaavu* (heat) any more in the body. There is some tiredness. [...] cold is there now ... everything heated is needed' (Hutter 1994: 188).

Other aspects of the birthing process may be seen in terms of their communicational content as well as their direct physiological effect. Thus the

Table 8.1 *Phases, activities and central concepts in a birthing process*

Phase	Humoral and diet issues	Physical location	Pollution and spirit danger issues	Ritual activities
1. Pregnancy	Woman is 'hot'; 'heating' foods avoided; woman often expected to reduce food consumption	Normal	Special care to avoid risk of pollution or spirit attack	Preparatory rite of passage in some cases (e.g., first birth in Tamil nadu)
2. Birth		Birthing room (*atul ghor*, etc.)	Birth seen as involving major pollution and risk of spirit attack	Ritual activity as needed to assist childbirth
3. Post-birth confinement (*narak ka samay*, etc)	Woman is 'cold'; she is kept warm; special 'heating' foods supplied; 'cooling' foods avoided	Birthing room (*atul ghor*, etc.)	Woman is at risk of spirit attack and is also dangerous to others; has to be confined	Ritual counter measures against possible attack (iron, amulets, etc.)
4. End of confinement (typically 5th or 6th day after birth, sometimes longer)		Birthing room (*atul ghor*, etc.)	Fate of child is determined by deity on preceding night	Rite of passage involving offerings to protective goddess of children (*Shashthi, Bemata, Shetigaava*, etc.)
5. Motherhood	Gradual return to normal diet and condition	Normal	Risk of spirit attack reduced but remains	Ritual counter measures (amulets, etc.) continue at lesser level

restrictions on the mother's mobility in the immediate post-birth period (the *narak ka samay* or 'hell time' of Chawla's *dais*) are routinely linked to her supposed extreme susceptibility to malevolent spirits (*bhut*, etc.) and other evil influences and also to the risk she poses to other people because of her polluted state. Concern with spirit-attack, 'evil eye', black magic and the like are a regular theme in accounts of birth in South Asia (e.g., Afsana and Rashid 2000: 28, van Hollen 2003: 136–137), and also underlie the extensive use of amulets, ritually empowered liquids and other protective devices (e.g., Rozario 1998: 145–147, van Hollen 2003: 136). Given this, it seems reasonable to assume that the post-birth restrictions have an effect on the mother and family's understanding of the situation as well as a direct physiological effect through the women's physical confinement to a limited space.

One might take this kind of analysis further. I am primarily interested here, however, in pointing out that there is both a physiological and a communicative aspect to what is going on, and that they are essentially inseparable. To put it in other terms, what is happening is happening to both mind and body together, or rather to the mind-body totality. It is that totality which is being formed and shaped, or rather which the new mother has to learn herself to form and shape.

Suppose now that we move to the alternative of biomedicalised birthing in a hospital – and we might consider here the typically depersonalised and heavily medicalised process of childbirth in many South Asian hospitals. Biomedical provision may be more appropriate in its own terms, for example, in the provision of proper diagnosis and hygiene, though one certainly cannot take this for granted (see, for example, Rozario 1995: 103–104), but it is alienated from the birthing woman and her family, owned by people who are typically very distant from her in culture, class and even language, and who are dismissive of the values held by her and her family (Jeffery et al. 1989: 115–118). Their procedures make very little sense to the birthing woman, except for the ubiquitous 'injections' and 'salines', which have been thoroughly incorporated into folk understandings of health and healing, if not necessarily in a way closely related to official biomedical perspectives. Above all, for most women, the hospital is a foreign and hostile place to be. Thus van Hollen comments in particular on women's fear of being alone in hospital:

> There is little doubt that the fear brought on from being alone in [large government] hospitals served to exacerbate the experience of the pain. So although women were frightened into silence [by the scolding of hospital staff], some could not control themselves, and many said there was a greater tendency towards panic in the hospital than at home (van Hollen 2003: 130).

Afsana and Rashid speak of how rural Bangladeshi women are intimidated by the hospital environment, with its threatening array of instruments, and cite the comment of one woman who shared the widespread fear of episiotomy, which can in fact have major consequences for a rural woman since it may limit her ability to perform household chores and lead to her body being labelled as 'defective':

> As soon as I entered the labour room, I closed my eyes in fear. I was too scared to think of the glittering instruments. I heard them talking about scissors. I was waiting and thinking to myself – when will they cut my vagina. Thank goodness, they didn't hurt me. Later on I heard they needed scissors to cut the umbilical cord. (Afsana and Rashid 2000: 34)

In a study from Indonesia, Hunter (2002) reports of a happy cooperation between tradition and modernity in a small local clinic where the staff were themselves local and sympathetic to the woman's concerns. But unfortunately such cases are exceptional for poor rural women in South Asia. Such women generally encounter the medical system in a hostile and painful manner when they are themselves in a state of medical crisis (e.g., Rozario 1995). In these situations, even if, for example, diet is 'healthy' in biomedical terms (and that is far from being certain), a lot of other things, at the cultural level, are not.

I would like us to remain aware that all along, in all these situations, 'traditional' or biomedical, both levels are operative on both sides. This is even more significant in situations of medical pluralism, where patients may be receiving biomedical treatment phrased primarily in physical and organic terms, and other forms of treatment that are phrased mostly in spiritual or other non-physiological terms. It is important to appreciate that in fact both kinds of 'treatment' are involved on both levels (body and spirit) and that the levels are in fact not ultimately separable. We really need a language that enables us to track things on both levels all the time.

All this is not to say that biomedicine does not have plenty to offer. But biomedicine in places like rural Bangladesh is often provided in an inadequate, ignorant and inappropriate manner, and is accompanied by the denial or exclusion of traditional supportive cultural practices. If the traditional procedures can have a positive 'placebo effect', biomedical practices may well have a negative one.

Where do we go from here? Perhaps we need to write new texts and manuals for Third World doctors (for all doctors, for that matter) that explicitly value and give presence to these issues as part of their training. Somehow, a better future for the birthing women of India and Bangladesh, and the health systems of the Third World more generally, needs to be built on a dual awareness, of the positive aspects of the traditional along with the positive aspects of what modernity has to offer.

Note

1. It is important not to overgeneralise. There are considerable variations between parts of Bangladesh and North India, and for that matter within communities. However, my point in this paper is less to do with the specific historically determined birth practices in particular

locations (see Rozario and Samuel 2002a for a variety of studies of this kind, and Samuel 2002 for some comments on differences between them) than with the general question of understanding of mind-body processes.

References

Afsana, K. and S.F. Rashid. 2000. *Discoursing Birthing Care: Experiences from Bangladesh*. Dhaka: University Press Limited.

Bateson, G. 1973. *Steps to an Ecology of Mind*. Frogmore: Paladin.

Chawla, J. 1994. *Childbearing and Culture: Woman-centred Revisioning of the Traditional Indian Midwife: The Dai as Ritual Practitioner*. New Delhi: Indian Social Institute.

——2002. '*Hawa, Gola* and Mother-in-law's Big Toe: On Understanding *Dais*' Imagery of the Female Body', in S. Rozario and G. Samuel (eds) *The Daughters of Hariti: Childbirth and Female Healers in South and Southeast Asia*. London and New York: Routledge, 147–162.

Hunter, C. 2002. 'Embracing Modernity: Transformations in Sasak Confinement Practices', in S. Rozario and G. Samuel (eds) *The Daughters of Hariti: Childbirth and Female Healers in South and Southeast Asia*. London and New York: Routledge, 279–297.

Hutter, I. 1994. *Being Pregnant in Rural South India: Nutrition of Women and Well-Being of Children*. Amsterdam: Thesis Publishers.

Jeffery, P., R. Jeffrey and A. Lyon. 1989. *Labour Pains and Labour Power: Women and Childbearing in India*. London: Zed Books.

Jeffery, P.M., R. Jeffery and A. Lyon. 2002. 'Contaminating States: Midwifery, Childbearing and the State in Rural North India', in S. Rozario and G. Samuel (eds) *The Daughters of Hariti: Childbirth and Female Healers in South and Southeast Asia*. London and New York: Routledge, 90–108.

Jeffery, R. and P.M. Jeffery. 1993. 'A Woman Belongs to Her Husband: Female Autonomy, Women's Work and Childbearing in Bijnor', in A.W. Clark (ed.) *Gender and Political Economy: Explorations of South Asian Systems*. Delhi: Oxford University Press, 66–114.

Kapferer, B. 1979. 'Mind, Self and Other in Demonic Illness: The Negation and Reconstruction of Self', *American Ethnologist* 6: 110–133.

——1983. *A Celebration of Demons: Exorcism and the Aesthetics of Healing in Sri Lanka*. Bloomington: Indiana University Press.

Kotalová, J. 1993. *Belonging to Others: Cultural Construction of Womanhood among Muslims in a Village in Bangladesh*. Uppsala University, distributed by Almqvist and Wiksell, Stockholm. (Acta Universitatis Upsaliensis. Uppsala Studies in Cultural Anthropology 19).

Laderman, C. 1987. 'The Ambiguity of Symbols in the Structure of Healing', *Social Science & Medicine* 24: 293–301.

Lamb, S. 2000. *White Saris and Sweet Mangoes: Aging, Gender, and Body in North India*. Berkeley, Los Angeles and London: University of California Press.

Lévi-Strauss, C. 1977 [1949]. 'The Effectiveness of Symbols', in C. Lévi-Strauss *Structural anthropology*. Vol. 1. Harmondsworth: Penguin, 186–206. [Originally published as 'L'efficacité symbolique,' in *Revue de l'Histoire des Religions* 135: 5–27.]

Manderson, L. 1981. 'Roasting, Smoking and Dieting in Response to Birth: Malay Confinement in Cross-Cultural Perspective', *Social Science & Medicine* 15B: 509–520.

Patel, T. 1994. *Fertility Behaviour: Population and Society in a Rajasthan Village.* Delhi: Oxford University Press.

Ram, K. 2001. 'Modernity and the Midwife: Contestations Over a Subaltern Figure, South India', in L.H. Connor and G. Samuel (eds) *Healing Powers and Modernity: Traditional Medicine, Shamanism, and Science in Asian Societies.* Westport, CT.: Bergin and Garvey, 64–84.

Rozario, S. 1995. 'Dai and Midwives: The Renegotiation of the Status of Birth Attendants in Contemporary Bangladesh', in J. Hatcher and C. Vlassoff (eds) *The Female Client and the Health-Care Provider.* Ottawa: International development Research Centre (IDRC) Books, 91–112.

——1998. 'The Dai and the Doctor: Discourses on Women's Reproductive Health in Rural Bangladesh', in K. Ram and M. Jolly (eds) *Modernities and Maternities: Colonial and Postcolonial Experiences in Asia and the Pacific.* Cambridge: Cambridge University Press, 144–176.

——2002. 'The Healer on the Margins: The *Dai* in Rural Bangladesh', in S. Rozario and G. Samuel (eds) *The Daughters of Hariti: Childbirth and Female Healers in South and Southeast Asia.* London and New York: Routledge, 130–146.

Rozario, S. and G. Samuel (eds) 2002a. *The Daughters of Hariti: Childbirth and Female Healers in South and Southeast Asia.* London and New York: Routledge.

——2002b. 'Tibetan and Indian Ideas of Birth Pollution', in S. Rozario and G. Samuel (eds) *The Daughters of Hariti: Childbirth and Female Healers in South and Southeast Asia.* London and New York: Routledge, 182–208.

Samuel, G. 1990a. *Mind, Body and Culture: Anthropology and the Biological Interface.* Cambridge and New York: Cambridge University Press.

——1990b. 'Mind, Body and Culture: A Brief Introduction', paper for seminar at Department of Anthropology, University of California, Berkeley, December 1990. E-text at http://users.hunterlink.net.au/~mbbgbs/Geoffrey/baglunch.html

——1999. 'Religion, Health and Suffering among Contemporary Tibetans', in J.R. Hinnells and R. Porter (eds) *Religion, Health and Suffering.* London and New York: Kegan Paul International, 85–110.

——2001a. 'Tibetan Medicine in Contemporary India: Theory and Practice', in L.H. Connor and G. Samuel (eds) *Healing Powers and Modernity in Asian Societies: Traditional Medicine, Shamanism and Science.* Westport, CT.: Bergin and Garvey (Greenwood Publishing), 247–268.

——2001b. 'The Effectiveness of Goddesses: An Interpretation of Discourse about Spirits', *Anthropological Forum* 11: 73–91.

——2002. 'Introduction', in S. Rozario and G. Samuel (eds) *The Daughters of Hariti: Childbirth and Female Healers in South and Southeast Asia.* London and New York: Routledge, 1–33.

Turner, V.W. 1968. *The Drums of Affliction: A Study of Religious Processes among the Ndembu of Zambia.* Oxford: Clarendon Press.

——1969. *The Ritual Process.* London: Routledge and Kegan Paul.

——1970. *The Forest of Symbols.* Ithaca, New York: Cornell University Press.

Unnithan-Kumar, M. 1999. 'Households, Kinship and Access to Reproductive Health Care among Rural Muslim Women in Jaipur', *Economic and Political Weekly* 34(10–11): 621–630.

——2002. 'Midwives among Others: Knowledges of Healing and the Politics of Emotions in Rajasthan, Northwest India', in S. Rozario and G. Samuel (eds) *The Daughters of Hariti: Childbirth and Female Healers in South and Southeast Asia.* London and New York: Routledge, 109–129.

van Hollen, C. 2002. '"Baby Friendly" Hospitals and Bad Mothers: Manoeuvring Development in the Post-Partum Period in Tamil Nadu, South India', in S. Rozario and G. Samuel (eds) *The Daughters of Hariti: Childbirth and Female Healers in South and Southeast Asia.* London and New York: Routledge, 163–181.

——2003. *Birth on the Threshold: Childbirth and Modernity in South India.* Berkeley, Los Angeles and London: University of California Press.

9

Self, Soul and Intravenous Infusion

Medical Pluralism and the Concept of *samay* among the Naporuna in Ecuador*

Michael Knipper

Medical practice among the Kichwa-speaking, native population of the lower Napo River in Ecuador, the Naporuna, appears to be a classical situation of contemporary medical pluralism with 'traditional medicine' (or 'ethno-medicine') and 'Western biomedicine' as its main elements. This article is about one specific aspect of the pluralistic medical practice of the Naporuna, which gained increasing importance for the medical anthropological fieldwork I conducted in this region from 1997 to 1999. The question I will focus on is how an indigenous concept, like the Kichwa-notion *samay*, shapes the perception of biomedical devices and services by Naporuna patients and their relatives.

In Kichwa-language dictionaries and related ethnographic writings, *samay* is usually translated as 'breath', 'respiration' or 'rest' (Orr and Wrisley 1965, Mugica 1979, Cordero 1992). Other, more extensive interpretations and my own observations suggest that the notion *samay* refers, at the same time, to a very broad and complex understanding of such diverse issues (from a 'Western' point of view) like 'soul' or 'soul substance', 'life force', 'personhood', the 'inner will' and something akin to the physical 'resistance' of a person (cf. Palacio 1992, Guzmán 1997, Macdonald 1999, Uzendoski 2000). A special relation to the realm of the so-called 'ethnomedical' beliefs, concepts or practices of the Naporuna or their Kichwa-speaking neighbours in adjacent regions of the Amazon is, however, generally not ascribed to this notion: Apart from a few references regarding *samay* in the context of shamanism and healing – for example, as 'the root of shamanic power'

(Uzendoski 2000: 73) or as a means to strengthen the 'soul' of an ill or otherwise weak person by giving him *samay* in form of breath over the head (Guzmán 1997: 48, Uzendoski 2000: 89) – ethnographic descriptions of *samay* ascribe little importance to this concept for the Naporuna's treatment and perception of disease. Despite this apparently insignificant relation between *samay* and any kind of health-related beliefs and practices – 'traditional' as well as 'modern' – a more detailed examination of this issue, which was inspired by some particular experiences with the pluralistic medical practice among the Naporuna, was able to disclose the great significance of the beliefs, experiences and practices related to *samay* for the perceptions of both local and biomedical healing practice by the Naporuna. Of crucial importance for this approach was the relation of *samay* with the analytical category 'self', which is understood as the culturally shaped conception of human beings as individual persons.

The analysis of *samay* presented in this paper was primarily stimulated by very pragmatic issues related to healthcare among the Naporuna. During my fieldwork, I worked both as a physician and as a medical anthropologist while conducting a study about the so-called indigenous disease category *mal aire* ('evil wind' or 'evil air', cf. Knipper 2003). As a result, this article also shows the insights to be gained if one combines various theoretical perspectives towards disease, health and healing – including critical approaches towards biomedicine and essentialist conceptualisations of issues like 'disease' or 'medicine' – with the pragmatic and therapeutic attitude of a health worker. As all the data and interpretations presented below are influenced by the double role I played among the Naporuna, they have to be preceded by some remarks on the particular fieldwork conditions and a reflection upon its main methodological consequences.

Fieldwork conditions and methodological remarks

I conducted my fieldwork in the region of the lower Napo River (see map, Figure 9.1) for a period of about twenty months between 1997 and 1999. While I was attending to patients, either alone or with indigenous community health workers in the small health posts of one of the Naporuna settlements along the river, I became an active part of the therapeutic pluralism in the region.

Communication took place mainly in Spanish and some in Kichwa. In these situations, the company of key informants and research assistants among the community health workers proved to be very helpful. They not only were able to provide me with detailed translations of Kichwa statements but also commented on and contradicted my interpretations and provisional conclusions.

The area of my study was the region between the provincial capital, Coca, and the Peruvian border at Nuevo Rocafuerte. The river provided the sole route of communication and transportation in the area. The distance between

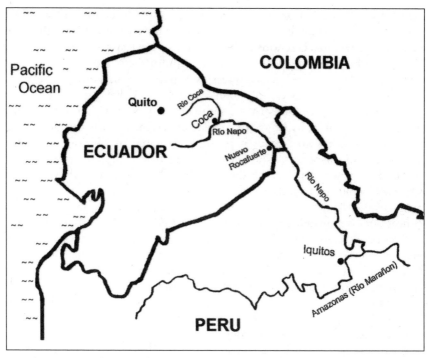

Figure 9.1 *Map showing fieldwork site: The region of the Lower Napo River, Ecuador*

Coca and Nuevo Rocafuerte is about 300km. In Coca and Nuevo Rocafuerte there are some hospitals, but the quality of attendance especially in the public hospital of the provincial capital is poor, and the private clinics are expensive. Occasional biomedical services are provided by the Ecuadorian army and oil companies, but the most reliable health service is supplied by the community health workers, nurses and physicians of a primary healthcare programme, which is carried out by the diocese of Aguarico and the Federation of the Naporuna Communities (FCUNA).

Regarding the methodological consequences of my engagement within the therapeutic pluralism of this region, I will mention here three basic points:[1] First, I got in touch with the patients and their families at a time when the disease outcome remained uncertain, when the interpretation of the case was still being negotiated and important decisions had to be made. In this moment, any specific disease condition appears very different from the retrospective view developed in an interview and from when the patient is already cured or deceased.

As a second point, in this moment of acute, threatening disease and subsequent actions, the biological aspects of the affliction – the ailments, the symptoms, the materially tangible signs – play a dominant role and can not be ignored. They definitely do not neutralise or extinguish other aspects, such as the social or the search for meaning. The physical and the social are not mutually exclusive categories: every bodily expression as well as the perception of material signs are culturally shaped. But the overwhelming presence of pain, blood and concrete suffering helps to avoid a merely 'aseptic' and predominantly theoretic perspective upon disease, healthcare and medical pluralism, where sickness appears to be a mainly socially or culturally defined issue and medical pluralism to be a problem of primarily theoretical and academic interest.

Third, I was able to observe the way people actually used my medical service in the everyday practice, how they explained to me, for example, their complaints, desires and priorities. In regard to the topic of medical pluralism, I could appreciate from a really well situated observation point the specific contexts in which people came to consult me as a physician (most of the time as the only physician on trips lasting one to two days) and in which they did not consult me. On several occasions, when I was present – in a household or at a public meeting, for example – and someone fell ill, no one asked me to help. And several times I was indeed asked to help, but not as a physician able to supply antibiotics, antimalarials, aspirin, other pills or a little surgery, but in a 'traditional' way: I was asked to blow tobacco smoke upon the ill person or to fan strong-smelling leaves over the patient in a group of about five or six persons, producing a wind that was supposed to cure. In these situations, I had the impression that for the Naporuna it was evident that biomedical aid was not necessary and that what was going on had nothing to do with my knowledge and experience as a physician. They were able to do me the great favour of perceiving me as a 'normal' person and not exclusively as a physician. I was happy and impressed. The 'biomedical doctor' did not disturb, and people did what they thought had to be done for the patient, independent of my presence. But I, from a methodological point of view, enjoyed the particular opportunity to observe how the people acted in situations when the two main elements of medical pluralism – local methods and biomedicine – were present and equally available. In other situations, the same people with often 'identical' problems (from my point of view: coincidence of symptoms, etc.) came to consult me, woke me up urgently at night or asked me to come to their homes to look after a patient. I remember even some cases, where I was initially asked to help by shaking leaves, and some hours or days later to provide biomedical medicines.

The most instructive and fruitful situations of my research have been those where I worked together with one of the 'indigenous healers', the *yachak*.[2] In such moments of combined treatment, I began to ask myself the questions which brought my attention to the notion of *samay*: How do people perceive my biomedical treatments? Why do they ask me for help and what do they expect? Their enigmatic decisions to ask or not, to explain their complaints or not, the words some patients used to describe their problems and expectations in my consultation office ('do you have injections?') and many other observations, made me think of the way they perceive biomedicine – a kind of perception, that did not coincide with mine. But what was the difference?

One of the key experiences that helped me develop a meaningful answer to this question was one of these 'bi-cultural' healing sessions. It was the story of the little girl Maria.[3] Apart from some hints in regard to the questions related to *samay* and the indigenous perception of healing, this case study also provides a vivid insight into the living conditions and the practical side of medical pluralism in the region.

Maria

I first remember meeting Maria, as she sat in her godparents' home, where I came to look in on her ill cousin. She was a five-year-old girl and lived with her parents about half an hour walking distance from where we lived in this Naporuna community. While her cousin was suffering from abdominal pain, Maria appeared to be well; thus I did not pay her any special attention. Like on other occasions when I was called to see a patient in a household, a *yachak* had also been sent for. While I examined the boy and talked to the old and experienced *yachak* Don Valentín, I saw Maria sitting in a corner of the house in front of Rodrigo, a relatively young *yachak* and apprentice of the former, who was slowly blowing tobacco smoke upon her head.

One day later, Maria and her parents came to my office. She was astonishingly pale and weak. I became a little bit nervous because my therapeutic possibilities were limited. But the family felt unable to undertake a trip to the hospital, which is about 150 kilometres down the river. I treated her with antiparasitic drugs and advised her parents immediately to take the girl to the hospital aboard any one of the commercial boats that travelled down the river every day. Only a few hours later, they again called and asked for my assistance, saying that Maria's condition was urgent. She was bleeding heavily from her gut and had fallen unconscious. At such a late hour on a dark, rainy afternoon in the Amazon, it was not possible to reach the hospital. So I sat half a day and a whole night together with Don Valentín at the girl's bedside. At the insistence of Maria's family, I put her on an intravenous infusion with a physiologically inadequate 10 per cent sugar solution, which I considered useless. I had no other infusion available because I had spent the last 'Ringer' solution on a patient bleeding from a considerable cut on his back a few days before. As the sugar solution slowly dripped into the vein of the barely respiring Maria, Don Valentín took his *aya waska* and began to sing the whole night long, quietly, softly but continuously. From time to time he interrupted his singing, illuminated the sugar-solution bottle with his electric torch and asked me: 'Does it go, Miguel?' Then, he went on singing and blowing tobacco smoke upon the girl. In this way, we spent the whole night.

In the early hours of the next morning, we managed to prepare a boat, to get gasoline and to take the trip to the hospital in Nuevo Rocafuerte. We arrived in the evening and the little girl survived with the help of oxygen, blood from her mother and drugs against the tropical malaria she had contracted and the intestinal parasites, which had penetrated her gut. The infusion I had given her during the night, from the physiological point of view, could not have had any major effect. And the 'unspecific' pharmacological effect, identified generally in a more or less disparaging way as the 'placeboeffect', may have been important but cannot explain sufficiently the impact of the intravenous infusion in this concrete situation. The significance of this chemically defined and industrially produced object of Western hospital-based medicine lies far beyond the realm of physiological knowledge and biomedical beliefs.

What is really interesting here is the meaning of the infusion for the Naporuna involved in Maria's disease history; for her parents, the relatives and friends present in the house as well as the *yachak*, the same people who had to convince me, the Western physician, to put the child on an infusion, which I myself considered as lamentably useless. The indigenous concepts relevant in this situation can further explain why people asked for both Don Valentín and me to help, and what they expected from our therapeutic efforts. Evidently, they did not distinguish between 'spirits' and 'soul loss' as regards Don Valentín and 'sugar solutions' and 'fluid replacement' while thinking about my biomedical efforts.

Possibly, during these extended moments at the bedside of the little girl, no one thought reflexively at all about these issues because they had other, more urgent preoccupations: Maria's life was in danger. Upon first observation, it is evident that the major motivation to combine both 'traditional' and 'Western' medicine was the urgent character of the problem and the uncertainty of its causes. Furthermore, both options were available: Valentín and I were present and respected by the people. But apart from the mere acknowledgement of the compatibility between different medical conceptions and therapeutic options as a matter of fact and of little concern for contemporary research (Miles and Leatherman 2003: 9), it remains interesting and relevant to look for positive statements to the question of *how* the integration of strange medical devices and practices succeed and *what* the relevant cultural patterns and perceptions are. The significance of the intravenous infusion in the situation described above had to do, in particular, with *samay* and the Naporuna's perception of body, self, soul and personality. Sugar solutions, blood pressure or renal circulation, in contrast, were as insignificant as clear-cut 'ethnomedical' beliefs with their narrow focus on local 'disease categories' and the supposed 'indigenous' elements of medical pluralism.

Samay

The following approximation of the indigenous concept of *samay* is based on translations and explanations found in Kichwa-language dictionaries and in ethnographic literature about Amazon Kichwa-speaking populations and, secondarily, other linguistic groups of this region. The search was focused especially on topics related to the perception of 'self', 'personhood' and allied topics. It was interesting to note that even among the heterogeneous Kichwa-speaking peoples, these concepts are not necessarily denominated with the same expression.[4] By the way, it was not intended to develop a complete and ultimate bibliography of this issue among indigenous groups in the Amazon. A third type of data are, finally, my personal observations during fieldwork.

According to relevant dictionaries of the Ecuadorian Kichwa language, the translation of *samay* generally consists in the notions 'breath' or 'respiration' (Orr and Wrisley 1965: 76, Mugica 1979: 106, Cordero 1992: 102) and 'rest' (Mugica 1979: 106, Cordero 1992: 102). The verb *samana*, accordingly, is translated as 'to breathe' and 'to rest'.

In various ethnographic studies, in contrast, the meaning of *samay* appears to be much more complex. The suggestions of Whitten (1985), Palacio (1992), Guzmán (1997) and the extensive work of Uzendoski (2000) coincided to a great extent with my own observations and proved to be especially useful for my interpretations.[5] Suggestions from other regions came principally from the very instructive contributions of Conclin and Morgan (1996), McCallum (1996) and Pollock (1996) to the ethnography of indigenous conceptions related to 'self', 'soul', 'personhood' and 'illness' among different native groups in the Amazon.

In synopsis, the different aspects of *samay*, which must be seen as linked and interwoven, can be described as follows:

In parts, *samay* coincides with the traditional Western and Christian notions of 'soul', though it must be differentiated from a concept expressed by the Kichwa word *aya*, which frequently becomes directly translated to the Spanish word *alma*. In contrast to *samay*, *aya* refers mainly to the soul of the deceased (cf. Mugica 1979: 83, Palacio 1992: 15–19, Uzendoski 2000: 75). To go further, it may be useful to describe *samay* as a kind of 'soul substance' (Uzendoski 2000: 71, 76) materially tangible in the 'breath' of a person and representing what is known in multiple cultural contexts all over the world as 'vital energy' or 'vital force' (Whitten 1985: 108). The 'inner power' of an individual person to live, to act and to realise his work belongs to the realm of *samay* (Guzmán 1997: 46), as well as a person's 'spiritual' and 'physical' resistance against any kind of disturbance (if one decides to introduce this problematic, but sometimes useful, dichotomy between the 'spiritual' and the 'physical' into analysis). It correlates to biomedically definable diseases as well as to the fright, for example, which follows the encounter with a spirit in the forest, or a condition like *mal aire* (Uzendoski 2000: 78).

Another aspect of *samay* comprises what can be described as 'personhood', the individual character, abilities and qualities of a human being (cf. Guzmán 1997: 46). The 'will' of a person, his ability to 'understand' and to 'comprehend' are part of this broad concept.

In addition to the various semantic and conceptual dimensions of *samay* described until now, both Guzmán (1997: 46–48) and Uzendoski (2000:

73–78) describe two further and especially important observations, which coincide with the observations of Conklin and Morgan (1996), McCallum (1996) and Pollock (1996) that relate to 'soul' and 'personhood' in other ethnic groups of the Amazon: they point out that *samay* is not a constant quality of the human being, but that it changes over time and can increase and decrease depending on the actual situation. Further, *samay* circulates among people: it can be transmitted among humans and non-humans and can be increased or reduced by the action of third parties, mainly by *yachaks*, spirits of the forest, mountains or rivers, or by the souls (*aya*) of ancestors. The *aya* are supposed to walk – for example after their funeral – through the forest or near the households. These two aspects, the dynamic and communicative qualities of *samay*, proved to be very instructive in relation to my own observations in the medical field.

I will conclude my description of *samay* with some examples, which I hope can link together the different aspects of *samay* mentioned above.

The most common and frequently described situation of 'filling up' *samay* is the preparation of a young individual to become a *yachak*. Here, the transmission of *samay* takes place when an old and powerful *yachak* blows his breath upon the head of the other person; thus the young receives the *samay* of the old so that he or she may one day become a *yachak* too. A further source of an especially powerful kind of *samay* for any *yachak* are the different 'spiritual beings' known by the Naporuna by the notion *supay*. The more or less voluntary encounter with a *supay* in the forest, for example, can result in the transmission of *samay* of extraordinary power and quality and can prompt the initiation of a career as *yachak* for a person who previously had not aspired this.

Another occasion of 'filling up' *samay* is directly after birth. When a child is born, it lives (it is breathing, moving, eating, crying, etc.) but it is weak and vulnerable. It is helpless, with little vital power and easily falls ill. Consequently, a newborn baby is supposed to have little and really weak *samay*. It is well known among the Naporuna that the first year of life is the most dangerous. For this reason, old people and sometimes a *yachak* blow upon the head of a newborn child. The breath in this situation is also called *samay*. Nowadays, this custom is losing importance and people associate 'blowing' upon a baby with the transmission of specialised *samay*, i.e., to prepare it to become *yachak*.

During the further life cycle of a person, when a child grows up and becomes an adult, personal *samay* is supposed to increase. The individual gains power, resistance and the ability to realise his or her life in a more and more autonomous way. Working, having a family and living in harmony with kith and kin are of overwhelming importance in becoming a 'person'. All this, as my informants told me, correlates to having a strong and resistant *samay*. But when disease befalls a person, *samay* decreases. He or she cannot work, cannot fulfil the obligations of reciprocity, social activities are interrupted or decrease and he or she is in danger of dying. Consequently, it is necessary to fill him up with new *samay*, with power and resistance. And so, every curative action of a *yachak*, when confronted by a serious or threatening illness consists of or is accompanied by the transmission of *samay*. No threatening disease is treated without blowing upon the ill person's head.

Normally, this responsibility falls upon a *yachak*. But if no one is available, any person with 'strong' *samay* can do so. And much like the breath of a *yachak*, blown upon the head of an ill or otherwise weak person, the liquid of the infusion bottle, which slowly dripped into Maria's vein and the coloured pills called 'vitamin compound tablets' or 'ferrous sulphate and folic acid dragees', prescribed by the physician for mothers feeling weak and tired, are understood to be a 'modern' kind of *samay*. And this indigenous perception is 'proven', when, for example, the intravenous infusion of an adequate solution strengthens a weak person, who from the biomedical point of view has suffered from dehydration. Similar situations are given day by day when young mothers or (generally as a consequence of intestinal parasites) anaemic children recover a few days after taking iron pills.

The actions and corresponding material objects introduced by the physician hold (or gain) indigenous meaning, which makes them 'useful' in a more than purely material or pragmatic way. People neither stop thinking when they are confronted with formerly unknown or strange methods of treating disease, nor do they passively adopt the biomedical theories and beliefs behind these objects and practices. And although Western biomedicine does not accept ideas like 'vital power', 'life force', *samay* or the Chinese *qi* as relevant for its theoretical models (cf. Kleinman 1995: 36), this by no means excludes patients (and even some practitioners) from considering this dimension when dealing with biomedical devices, services, institutions and staff.

Conclusions

On several occasions, the interpretation of *samay*, as described above, proved to be useful to my work as a physician among the Naporuna. Recognising *samay* as a highly flexible indigenous category of perception, which comprises such apparently disparate issues like 'breath', 'respiration', 'soul', 'personhood' and 'vital force', considerably improved my ability to communicate in the quotidian cooperation with patients, their relatives and *yachak*. It provided me with a suitable explanation for the, at a superficial glance, surprising and apparently 'irrational' way the Naporuna employ biomedical devices and services – a problem physicians, medical anthropologists and other strangers also have to face in regions other than the Amazon.

With this outcome, the major goal of my study was achieved: The health related decisions and the behaviour of Naporuna patients and practitioners no longer appeared to be as striking and astonishing as they did initially. I was able to understand patients' complaints better than before and to explain them my own opinions and interpretations in respect to a concrete disease or health problem in a more appropriate way.

Through my active involvement in the health-seeking process, with nearly daily contacts with patients and different kinds of 'local healers', the apparently clear-cut boundaries between different 'medical systems' lost all of their seductive power. In the real life of patients as well as practitioners, this distinction is of so little importance that it can be neglected without problems.[6] Dependant upon the aims of each study, it may or may not be useful to acknowledge the theoretical models and categories about medical pluralism, which have been developed to approach the structural and political aspects of this ubiquitous phenomenon. The application of analytic categories like 'medical system' or 'practitioner systems' for example, which proved to be helpful and instructive in some occasions, can be misleading and confusing in others. And even the analytic tool called 'explanatory model', which I used widely in the first months of my fieldwork, turned out to be too unspecific. The usual methodological devices to elicit an indigenous Explanatory Model (as, for example, the questions proposed by Kleinman 1980: 106), proved to be too narrow to grasp meaning and to develop appropriate interpretations in the face of the observations I made (and the answers I got) at the Napo River.

To understand the disease-related concepts and behaviours of the Naporuna, it was necessary to relate them to a non-medical concept (*samay*) and to overcome the nearly instinctively made distinction between 'local' and 'Western' medicine. It was astonishing that all those aspects of the indigenous culture, which proved to be relevant in the course of this study, by no means fit into any kind of ('ethno-') medical categories and even lost this character if it had been assumed before. *Samay,* for example, is not an ethnomedical notion and any attempt to develop such an interpretation would result in a crude medicalisation of indigenous terms. Even notions like *mal aire* or the well-known *susto,* widely recognised as 'ethnomedical' notions of Latin America, could not be considered in a predominantly 'medical' way (cf. Knipper 2003). Among the Naporuna, these terms refer to a much broader set of experiences, knowledge and practice than those related to disease and health. In daily life, they are not used to describe mutually exclusive categories for the interpretation and denomination of health problems, and the related concepts have just as little importance for the choice (or rejection) of a special kind of treatment. As a consequence, there remained little support for any 'medically' biased classification of these notions.

Looking back to the beginning of my work with the Naporuna, the thought of ever relating such strange things like 'self', 'soul' and 'intravenous infusions' at that time seemed entirely absurd. But my attempt to understand what people did with, and thought of, my simple (and mainly biologically defined) work as a physician, brought me to this point. I must stress the impact of the methodology as an important determinant of the surprising outcome of my study. Far beyond the theoretical considerations mentioned above, which although very important, easily got out of sight during daily fieldwork, the inductive character of my approach was responsible, to a considerable extent, for my results: I used the different techniques of gathering and analysing data with the explicit aim of eliciting comprehensible 'local' domains of meaning, knowledge and practice. With time (which is a very important factor!) and as a consequence of the repeated and critical reconsiderations of my contradictory and disconnected findings, insights into the importance of the notion *samay* arose during my field observations. The analytic category 'self', finally, did the same among the repertoire of my own intellectual devices.

Notes

* I thank the editors of this volume, Helle Johannessen and Imre Lázár, as well as Volker Roelcke and Sahand Boorboor, for their very useful comments on earlier versions of this paper.
1. For a similar view on the specific 'bias' of anthropological research conducted by physicians, cf. Bolton 1995.
2. The Kichwa notion *yachak* is derived from the word *yachana*, which can be translated as 'to know'. The *yachak* are 'those who know' and their competence extends to a wide range of problems, from attending ill people to explaining disease, misfortune, etc. They achieved this via their connection to, and influence upon, the beings of the non-visible world, which is made possible, among other things, by the consumption of the drug called *aya waska*.
3. All the individual names are changed.
4. And sometimes it remains open, if the notion *samay* actually does not exist or is unknown among the particular Kichwa-speaking Indians described in some ethnographic studies, or if it was simply neglected in the course of the related investigation. This is the case, for example, in the early work of Whitten (1976) as well as in the books of Iglesias (1989) and Kohn (1992).
5. To a minor extent my research coincides with the writings of Whitten (1976), Hudelson (1987), Iglesias (1989) and Muratorio (1998).
6. In my experience, the only group of local actors which really pay attendance to this classification, are those 'traditional healers' engaged in the development of a professionally organised 'traditional indigenous medicine'.

References

Bolton, J. 1995. 'Medical Practice and Anthropological Bias', *Social Science & Medicine* 40(12): 1655–1661.
Conklin, B.A. and L.M. Morgan. 1996. 'Babies, Bodies, and the Production of Personhood in North America and a Native Amazonian Society', *Ethos* 24(4): 657–694.
Cordero, L. 1992 [1895]. *Diccionario Quichua-Castellano y Castellano-Quichua.* Quito: Corporación Editora Nacional.
Guzmán, M. 1997. *Para que la yuca beba nuestra sangre. Trabajo, género y parentesco en una comunidad quichua de la Amazonia Ecuatoriana.* Quito: Ed. Abya-Yala / CEDIME.

Hudelson, J.E. 1987. *La cultura quichua en transición. Su expansión y desarrollo en el Alto Amazonas.* Guayaquil / Quito: Museo Antropológico del Banco Central del Ecuador / Abya-Yala.

Iglesias, G. 1989. *Sacha Jambi. El uso de las plantas en la medicina tradicional de los Quichuas del Napo.* Quito: Ediciones Abya-Yala.

Kleinman, A. 1980. *Patients and Healers in the Context of Culture. An Exploration of the Borderland between Anthropology, Medicine and Psychiatry.* Berkeley: University of California Press.

———1995. *Writing at the Margin: Discourses between Anthropology and Medicine.* Berkeley: University of California Press.

Knipper, M. 2003. *Krankheit, Kultur und medizinische Praxis. Eine medizinethnologische Untersuchung zu 'mal aire' im Amazonastiefland von Ecuador.* Münster: Lit (Spanish version will be available in summer / fall 2005 in Quito, Ecuador: Ediciones Abya Yala / CICAME).

Kohn, E.O. 1992. *La cultura médica de los Runas de la región amazónica ecuatoriana.* Quito: Ediciones Abya-Yala.

Macdonald, T. Jr. 1999. *Ethnicity and Culture amidst New 'Neighbors'. The Runa of Ecuador's Amazon Region.* Boston: Allyn and Bacon.

McCallum, C. 1996. 'The Body that Knows: From Cashinahua Epistemology to a Medical Anthropology of Lowland South America', *Medical Anthropology Quarterly* 10(3): 347–372.

Miles, A. and T. Leatherman. 2003. 'Perspectives on Medical Anthropology in the Andes', in J.D. Koss-Chioino, T. Leatherman and C. Greenway (eds) *Medical Pluralism in the Andes.* London and New York: Routledge, 3–15.

Mugica, C. 1979. *Aprenda el Quichua. Gramática y vocabularios.* Pompeya (Ecuador): Ediciones CICAME.

Muratorio, B. 1998. *Rucuyaya Alonso y la historia social y económica del Alto Napo 1850–1950.* (2. ed.) Quito: Ediciones Abya-Yala.

Orr, C. and B. Wrisley. 1965. *Vocabulario Quichua del Oriente del Ecuador.* Quito: ILV (= Serie de vocabularios indígenas 11).

Palacio, J.L. 1992. *Muerte y Vida en el Río Napo.* Pompeya (Ecuador): Ediciones CICAME.

Pollock, D. 1996. 'Personhood and Illness among the Kulina', *Medical Anthropology Quarterly* 10(3): 319–341.

Uzendoski, M.A. 2000. 'The Articulation of Value among the Napo Runa of the Upper Ecuadorian Amazon'. Unpublished Ph.D. Thesis, University of Virginia.

Whitten, N.E. 1976. *Sacha Runa. Ethnicity and Adaptation of Ecuadorian Jungle Quichua.* Urbana: University of Illinois Press.

Whitten, N.E. 1985. *Sicuanga Runa. The Other Side of Development in Amazonian Ecuador.* Urbana: University of Illinois Press.

10

Experiences of Illness and Self
Tamil Refugees in Norway Seeking Medical Advice

Anne Sigfrid Grønseth

This paper focuses on links between medical pluralism, refugee health issues and forms of healing that together are seen through a lens of self and well-being as part of a process of embodiment. The study is concerned with individual Tamil persons that experience and embody a dramatic social and cultural change that challenge questions of illness and healing as these are interconnected to constitutions of identity and personhood. The investigation was conducted among Tamil refugees in Norway who make use of and negotiate between various medical approaches to health and well-being. I see Tamils' quest for well-being as broadly defined and embedded in social and religious relations. From this perspective, health and healthcare are not limited to the arena of interaction between doctor and patient, but involve a variety of coping strategies among the 'normal' Tamil population. Also, the perspective of well-being acknowledges the traditional perspectives of medical pluralism (Loudon 1976, Kleinman 1980, Jacobson-Widding and Westerlund 1989, Samson 1999, and others), and opens for less recognized aspects such as social or communitarian practices. Additionally, I seek to avoid the difficulties related to the often-used concepts of disease, illness and disorder (Kleinman 1980, Hahn 1984, and others).

The Tamil refugees in Norway tend to experience various diffuse aches and pains, which brings them to the local health centre for consultations. At the health centre they meet physicians and staff that are trained in biomedicine and as such are focused on understanding illness and health as result of individual and physical conditions. Accordingly, Tamils are met with an understanding of their suffering which separates body from soul and individual from social. Among Tamils such distinctions are not common and seem to produce uncertainty and confusion about the Norwegian health treatment. Such confusion is seen as related to Tamils' familiarity with Ayurvedic medicine and other ways of understanding well-being and sickness. Health and well-being are in profound and various ways connected to ideas and social practices in constructions of person and self. This essay will not explore different constructions of person and self as such. Rather, I suggest that when Tamils are forced to reorient themselves and negotiate in a radically new social and cultural world, this might be seen to enforce a deep insecurity in personal as well as group identity.

Looking into how Tamils' aches and pains may be related to a wider social world, I will explore an approach that collapses the Cartesian dichotomy of body and soul. By opening for an active perceptive body (Jackson 1989, Merleau-Ponty 2002) and seeing the self as an orienting point of 'being in the world' (Csordas 1994), I argue that Tamils embody ongoing social experiences which tend to produce diffuse enduring pains and fatigue. At one level, one may understand the pains as a bodily experience of social devaluation and stigmatisation (Goffman 1961, Bauman 1995). On another level, one may see the Tamils as living in a tension in which the self is forced to reorient itself in the world and thereby challenge habituated (Bourdieu 1989) patterns of how to constitute oneself as a worthy social person.

By the above-mentioned perspectives, I aim to address three aspects within a plurality of medical approaches that may be seen to exist among the Tamils. First, the Tamils seek advice at the local health centre. Second, the Tamils tend to reconstruct bits and pieces of familiar and traditional healing practices. These two aspects are situated within the traditionally recognised forms of medical pluralism that may be seen as reductive as they relate to the idioms of illness and disease. By the third and last aspect, I seek to transgress the boundaries between the normal and pathological as well as personal and social problems. Thus, I aim to open for perspectives that bring light to Tamils' healing forms and practices as part of a social or communitarian context, often overlooked within studies of medical pluralism.

Below I will shortly introduce the thematic context for this study and place of fieldwork. This is followed by two cases, which both in their own way are meant to illustrate Tamils' use of various medical approaches and how these together may be seen related to Tamils' experience of vast social, cultural changes. The following section looks into how Tamils' quest for healing and well-being in Arctic Harbor may be seen to generate new social and religious practices. Further, I suggest an analysis that aims to grasp how social experiences may be seen to confront and challenge Tamils' unconscious patterns and practices that provide a sense of self and person, and thus well-being.

Context of fieldwork

I was introduced to the field of Tamil refugees and issues of health and well-being during my work as a consultant with the Psychosocial Team for Refugees in Northern Norway. My colleagues referred to many doctors' and clinicians' reports on their difficulties in diagnosis and concern regarding the Tamil refugees. Several health workers expressed worry for the probability of Tamil suicides. I was never told of any such tragedy, but the possibility was discussed as part of a more general concern for Tamils' health and patterns of sickness. Since the medical and psychiatric approaches to many Tamils' complaints and symptoms did not prove adequate or sufficient I was encouraged to approach the situation from a social perspective. After a few years of shorter field visits,[1] in September 1999 I was able to start a year's fieldwork among the Tamil refugees in one of the small fishing villages.[2]

Data for this article were produced over a period of four years (1996–2000) during which, for the first three years I was employed as a consultant with the Psychosocial Team for Refugees in Northern Norway.[3] By the fall of 1999[4] I was able to conduct one year's fieldwork and concentrate my investigation on a community study based in Arctic Harbor.[5] This gave an opportunity for a closer focus on social aspects of health and well-being; raising issues related to concepts such as identity, community and nationhood (Daniel and Knudsen 1995, Buijs 1996, Jenkins 1996, Daniel 1997).

Arctic Harbor is situated on a small fiord by the Barents Ocean, with open sea all the way to the North Pole. Looking south, flat mountains rise from the sea leading into the Finnmarksvidda.[6] During the few months of summer the temperature rarely rises above twenty degrees C (sixty-eight degrees F), there is barely any vegetation except the vulnerable bushes and flowers in some of the houses' gardens. As winter sets in, cold blizzards shovel snow up along the buildings making it difficult and sometimes impossible to open the front door. Every now and then the roads as well as the small airport are closed down, leaving the little community isolated from hospital and other crucial services. From June until August the sun shines both day and night until it gradually disappears all together below the horizon from November until February.

Arctic Harbor offers well-paid jobs and good housing.[7] With only very few exceptions, all the Tamils are employed, in the traditionally women's low status job, as 'cutters' in the fishing industry. Many Tamils experience that they represent a group, which is not wanted in Arctic Harbor, and express daily experiences of degradations and humiliation. Tamils often report that they feel perceived by the local community only as 'black faces' or 'refugees' with no passage into the local social life. Together, one might say that the Tamils as a group experience a double stigmatisation; as low-status workers and as black Tamil refugees.

The Tamils tend to keep to themselves and have established a well-functioning Local Tamil Association that arranges a broad spectrum of social and religious activities. Although the Tamil population is well integrated into the local (and national) economy, they are socially and culturally segregated. They rarely mix with the locals. Nevertheless, some Tamils express a wish to live in small places such as Arctic Harbor because these places offer a well-paid job, a close network among the Tamils and a local Tamil Association providing an experience of social security and cultural continuity.

Every day and every minute Tamils in Arctic Harbor are confronted with questions of old and new ways of doing things that challenge them in the process of re-establishing a Tamil community and identity in exile. Tamil refugees in Arctic Harbor are not only deprived from the familiar Sri Lankan Tamil home-world, but are also confronted with a new and unknown Norwegian home-world which demands new ways of experiencing themselves as persons. Tamils meet such demands in contexts such as at work, in education and language training. Tamils are challenged to express and behave in a manner that corresponds with what may very roughly be described as Norwegian and Western ideas of 'the person' as comparably a more autonomous individual that seeks personal self-realisation, rather than a more dependent individual emphasising the fulfillment of collective interests (see Geertz 1973, Marriot 1976 and others). When meeting Norwegians, Tamils are often by way of questions and conversations indirectly expected to pursue self-interests and take part in skiing, hiking, solitary walks, food-diets and other typical Norwegian activities that are unfamiliar for most Tamils (see also Grønseth 1997, 2001).

Though meeting such demands in various contexts, they are maybe more precarious within the health arena. Questions of health and well-being are deeply connected with how one may experience one's self as a whole social and moral person. Considering the immense changes Tamil refugees are confronted with, my interest is not here focused on social construction of person and self, but more on understanding how Tamil selves seems to orient themselves and negotiate in the new social and cultural world. Opening for an actively perceptive human body one may see Tamils' complaints not only as individual somatisation but also as collective social experiences of 'being in the world' that are perceived and expressed by individual bodies. As part of Tamils' experiences and negotiations within issues of health and well-being Tamils struggle to comply with the Norwegian healthcare system. Simultaneously, the Tamils also may be seen to re-create old ways that within the radical new environment may generate whole new meanings that can be seen as part of a plural and flexible approach to practices that aim at healing and prosperity.

In the following, I document medical pluralism with two examples of different healing practices. The cases are contextualised and described within the realm of experience and daily life. To present the cases as dissected from everyday life experiences would be artificial as Tamils' healing and medical practices must be seen as closely interconnected with the challenges of day-to-day living. Analytically, the cases give examples of how Tamils' reconstruct fragments of Ayurvedic and traditional Tamil healing as well as creations of communitarian healing. The first case gives an example of how the Tamils struggle to reconstruct bits and parts of familiar traditional Tamil healing practices. The second case gives a detailed description of a child's birthday party and shows how the need of 'being together' may provide crucial healing aspects. The two cases together illustrate how questions of healing and well-being in various ways are related to questions of group and personal identity that are part of habituated patterns in the self's perception and orienting capacity of 'being in the world'.

Pillai and Padimini: 'I only know that sometimes a sickness makes you too hot or too cold. What can I do?'

One morning I visited the house of Pillai and Padimini. Pillai said he had been sick for one week and that the doctor had only told him to keep indoors and take fever reducing tablets if necessary. I asked how he felt about the Norwegian doctors and Pillai said:

> The problem is that Norwegian doctors only see my body and organs. They don't see my person. Very often doctors do nothing. We feel very uncertain. Padimini has prepared foods for me that should cool me down, but we don't know the effect of Norwegian foods. We have herb mixtures that are good when you are too hot, so I take some of it. Padimini gives me massage with oil that she brought with her when she came from Sri Lanka. It makes me feel very good. I relax and feel a refreshment.

Padimini joined into the discussion and told me that she had tried the same oil on Segar to reduce his rash. Padimini repeated Pillai's saying that 'the Norwegian health workers do nothing'. Also, Padimini took care to give Pillai a diet of vegetables and fish, and avoiding citrus fruits. She showed me that beneath Segar's clothing she had tied a new blessed string around his waist. Padmini said that she felt very insecure and preyed to the gods that they must protect and comfort the family.

Padimini and Pillai continued to tell me that they felt helpless in dealing with the family's various illnesses. On the one hand, they consult the Norwegian doctors and often find the help offered difficult to understand. Sometimes they come home with tablets they do not use. They said that they feel insecure about the effect. On the other hand, they try to deal with the illness within a frame of Tamil traditional healing, mainly based on Ayurvedic approaches. When I asked if they could tell me more about Tamil healing, Pillai explained to me that it was not easy to talk about this. He said: 'I can't explain how it works. It's just something we are accustomed to.' Padimini said that the family in Sri Lanka sometimes sent them mixtures and oils they used in various situations. She told me that towards the end of her pregnancy Padimini's mother had made sure to send her an Ayurvedic mixture of twenty-one distinct herbs. Padimini explained that after birth the uterus has sores along the side that needs to be healed. This mixture is meant to help the healing process. Padimini continued to tell me that in her family her mother often visited the temples and also sometimes an astrologer to consult on the family's health and well-being. While Padimini spoke she emphasised her uncertainty in dealing with health and illness when living in Norway:

> You know, when we use specific foods, herbs, mixtures and such, it's not something we talk about. I don't know how to explain. I only know that sometimes a sickness makes you too hot or too cold. So, you need to make food and use mixtures that will bring you back in balance. At home in Sri Lanka, many people know what to do. There's always someone to ask. When you visit the Tamil doctor you always get some pills, maybe herb mixtures and prescriptions for a diet. Sometimes the doctor gives you advice for meditation and oils to be used in massage. Here, the doctor doesn't want to know our problems and give no advice and no pills. They can't cure our difficulties. It's very hard. I've no one to ask and talk with.

Birthday party: 'We must be together and avoid difficulties'

Shortly after Bavishan and Geetha were reunited in Arctic Harbor, Bavishan became severely sick. He was hospitalised and on sick-leave for several months. Geetha turned to the gods for help and guidance. She put on a protective amulet that her sister had sent after visiting a religious healer. Every day Geetha prayed intensely to the gods that her husband must recover and she took special care to pay her due respect to the gods. Even though she felt very lonely and longed for the temples and family at home, she felt that her prayers were heard as Bavishan slowly recovered. Due to the timing of the unfortunate sickness, the local Tamil community perceived Geetha as a 'bearer of bad luck'. Geetha felt bad and was troubled by extensive headaches, dizziness and fatigue. She visited the local doctor but did not find the help and comfort that she needed. Geetha said:

> The doctors don't understand my problems. They only see my body and do tests. They don't help me.

When Bavishan and Geetha some time later were planning their youngest daughter's second birthday, they knew that most Tamil families were ambivalent to them and avoided contact. Thus, Bavishan and Geetha did not expect many guests. They acknowledged with regret that the stigma of Geetha being a 'bearer of bad luck' still hung over the family. Geetha said that she would not ask any of the other ladies to help her. She explained that she does not like the other women's talk. They talk too much and it easily evolves into difficulties between the ladies. When I inquired further, she only repeated:

> It's difficult. The ladies are nice, but I don't like their talk. There are many problems.

A few days later I came over in the morning to help her make the sweets and spicy crisps. We peeled almonds, melted sugar, boiled milk, ground different kinds of peas, blended flour, chopped onions and chili and stirred and baked for hours. Upon the day of the birthday I arrived in the afternoon. In the small entrance hall the candles were lighted and there was a lovely aroma of incense. In the sitting room, the room was beautifully decorated with silk flowers, a banner saying 'Thanuisha, 2 years, 10th March 2000', and a wonderful birthday cake made as a clown. The family was busily showering and dressing for the occasion. Then, we all ventured upstairs to the household shrine and did our puja-service and brought offering to the gods.

As the guests arrived, they were served a plate with a taste of all the foods. Time passed and the first guests started to return home while others were arriving. At about eight o'clock in the evening almost all the guests were new guests. All together, more or less twenty-five families visited. By the end of the evening, I asked Geetha how the party had been for her, and she replied:

I'm happy we made so much food. I didn't expect so many to come. It's good. So many came and ate our food. I'm very happy. Some of the women aren't nice, but it was a good party.

The next few days, a topic of interest during my various visits to Tamil families was to go through the names of those who were there and who where not. Obviously, the list of who was there gave interesting information about the social relations among the Tamils. But as Bavishan pointed out:

Living in Arctic Harbor we need to be together. At birthday, my house is open for everyone. But, also I know that not everyone will come. It's difficult. I can't choose my friends and I must be with people that I don't want to be with. Sometimes I'm happy to see someone come that I thought wouldn't come and sometimes families come that I don't want to be with. It's like this when we don't live at home. We must be together and avoid difficulties.

By way of exploring the various medical and health promoting approaches Tamils practice in the above cases, I will draw attention to how they in divers ways seem to relate to Tamil experiences of self and person. First, I present an analysis that looks into how Tamils strive to reconstruct Tamil traditional Ayurvedic healing as well as social and religious practices that enforce well-being and affluence. Here, I draw attention to healing not only as part of a specific medical approach, but also an important aspect within community and religious practices. Second, I suggest that the healing potential in community and religious practices may be grasped by looking into what may be seen as tensions in themes of self and personhood that are forced from a field of doxa into opinion (Bourdieu 1989). Understanding Tamils' diffuse aches and pains as part of tensions in habituated patterns for experiencing identity and well-being connects to how Tamils might be seen to seek cure and comfort within a plurality of health promoting practices.

Healing in religious and community experiences

Tamils' experience of the encounter with Norwegian health personal may be seen to generate confusion and vulnerability regarding personal identity. That many Tamils use fragments of Tamil traditional and Ayurvedic medical practices may be seen to reduce the occurrence of uncertainty and insecurity regarding self and person. This may be seen in the cases of Geetha and of Pillai and Padimini. Geetha says 'the doctors don't understand my problems' and is puzzled that the Norwegian doctors have no treatment. Pillai and Padimini both say: 'the Norwegian health workers do nothing'. Pillai expresses the comfort and support he experiences when Padimini gives him massage with oil from Sri Lanka. He says: 'It makes me feel very good. I relax and feel a refreshment.' Such statements may be seen to indicate a trust and comfort related to Ayurvedic medicine that fit with Tamil ways of experiencing themselves as body and person. Albeit, the themes of self and person are not always explicitly expressed, the Ayurvedic idioms of sickness also include ways of perceiving and conceptualising experiences of oneself as a social and moral person. Even though Geetha, Padimini and Pillai are not able to visit a Tamil Ayurvedic doctor or other traditional healers, they seem to experience confidence and comfort when making use of Ayurvedic medicine, diverse mixtures, oils and amulets. Thus, it seems that one may grasp a crucial aspect of Tamils' relation to health and cure when one considers how various traditional healing remedies supply a context of meaning that match to Tamil ways of experiencing themselves as being a person.

Padimini says that in Norway 'there's no one to ask and talk with'. The situation of not having anyone to discuss with is two-fold. It may be seen to refer to not being able to discuss matters of importance with the Norwegian doctor, but also to not have other Tamils whom one might discuss illness with. When at home in Sri Lanka, they are accustomed to treat various illnesses with specific foods, herbs and mixtures. How these prescriptions are interconnected and become potent for healing is not part of most Tamils' skills and knowledge. Generally, the Tamils tend to have only vague ideas about healing as a process in which one seeks to bring balance between concepts of 'hot' and 'cold'. How such a balance is achieved is only partly and vaguely known, especially among the rather young people that make the large majority of the Tamil refugees in Norway and Arctic Harbor. As Padimini says: 'At home in Sri Lanka, many people know what to do. There's always someone to ask… [In Arctic Harbor] it's very hard. I've no one to ask and talk with'. Still, the presented cases illustrate how many Tamils seek to reconstruct parts and fragments of Ayurvedic approaches together with other traditional healing practices. Geetha, Pillai and Padimini, as many other Tamils, refer to various herb mixtures, oils and attempts to construct beneficial diets while seeking to monitor a balance between hot and cold, and thus good health.

Considering the Tamils' fragmented use of Ayurvedic and traditional healing approaches, one might conclude that what the Tamils are searching for may not be the remedies in themselves, but the context of meaning and social relations that they provide. Tamil medicine is part of Tamil everyday life including Hindu life-philosophy and idioms of sickness that is closely connected to ideas of body, self and personhood, and as such supplies a context of meaning. Simultaneously, Tamils in Arctic Harbor who receive medical and health promoting remedies from friends, family and kin experience themselves as part of relations that are precarious for a sense of self, person and well-being. Thus, Tamils may be seen to search for healing, health and well-being not only by medical solutions, but also within religious and social relations that supply experiences of community and personhood.

Looking into the case of the birthday party one might see how Tamil health promoting practices not only includes fragments of Ayurvedic medicine, but also a search for community and religious experiences. This case shows how Geetha, who is considered to be a 'bearer of bad luck' and avoided by the Tamils, is brought together with others in the Tamil community. Geetha experiences various pains and symptoms such as headaches, dizziness and fatigue, but the Norwegian doctor finds no physical or organic explanation. In her despair, Geetha turns with intensified urge to the gods. Sharing parts of her everyday life, I was attuned to an engaged and empathic mode of insight, which enabled me to sense some of her aloneness and despair connected to her statement during the preparations for the birthday party: 'It's difficult. The ladies are nice, but I don't like their talk'.

Even though Geetha experiences great disturbances and tensions in being alone and avoided by the other Tamils, she also finds moments of joy and relief. In spite of the household altar not being as potent and comforting as the statues at the Hindu temples at home, she feels some comfort and support when worshiping the gods in the new setting of Arctic Harbor. Geetha even experienced what she described as 'the gods' mercy' when her husband recovered and returned home from the hospital. Considering her socially stigmatised position, Geetha did not care to (or dare to) ask the other Tamil women to help her prepare the foods for the party. Geetha and Bavishan did not expect many families to attend, but still they made enough for more than the double number of guests than they anticipated would come. Making everything ready for the party, Geetha was busy for many days with planning, organising and cooking. It was as though she wanted the family to appear at their best at this social occasion. When the party was finishing Geetha says: 'I didn't expect so many to come. It's good. So many came and ate our food. I'm very happy.' It was as if Geetha harvested the fruits of her effort. In light of Geetha's suffering of being labelled as a 'bearer of bad luck', one may consider the birthday party as an event of healing. Geetha may be seen as embraced by the Tamil community and as such she experienced relief and happiness. The birthday party provided a moment in which Geetha was part of relations that are crucial for her experience of self and personhood. Nevertheless, both Geetha and Bavishan not only emphasise the need to be together, but also acknowledge that there are some families (and women) they do not want to be with. Notwithstanding, Bavishan concludes: 'It's like this when we don't live at home. We must be together and avoid difficulties.'

The above references to Geetha's religious practices and the birthday party, as well as other aspects in the presented cases, together illustrate how Tamils in Arctic Harbor might be seen as stretched and pulled in new and different directions regarding questions of self-identity. Tamils may be seen as experiencing a pain of tensions enforced by great cultural and social changes. When consulting Norwegian healthcare workers, they are confronted with new and Norwegian local ways of constructing self and personhood. In addition, the Tamils are searching for ways to reconstruct and create new medical as well as social and religious practices that provide healing, well-being and experiences of self and personhood. Together, the Tamils may be seen to live in a tension of changes that stretches and enforces new ways of experiencing themselves as persons. In the following section, I look further into how one may see the handling of questions regarding self and person as part of Tamils' search for well-being and ways of healing.

Living between distinct worlds: healing and self

Tamils in Arctic Harbor may be seen as living in a tension between two home-worlds. One is the familiar Tamil home-world, which they have left but seek to reconstruct in bits and pieces. The other is the new and unknown surrounding Norwegian home-world in which they have settled and seek to learn about in parts and wholes. As previously mentioned, each one of the home-worlds represent distinct and different ways of constituting what may be termed as selfhood and social person (see Geertz 1973, Rosaldo 1980, Morris 1994, Lutz 1998). Studies of self and personhood among peoples in India and South Asia commonly emphasise an understanding of the individual as part of a greater social whole dependent on social and religious relations as elements in a socio-centric construction of self-identity (see Marriot 1976, Dumont 1980, Mines 1988, Kakar 1997). Classically, such an understanding of self and person is opposed to a Western idea of the self as an autonomous, inner authentic unit in an ego-centric construction of selfhood (Geertz 1973, Giddens 1991). Such oppositions in constructions of self and person must be seen as the far ends of a continuum where peoples and individuals move along the axis in respect to distinct situations and contexts.

Questions of self and person are not commonly reflected upon, but are habituated and taken for granted. As Tamils are torn out of their habituated everyday life, they are forced to reorient and negotiate new ways of being a social person. What has earlier been part of a doxic field is brought into a field of opinion (Bourdieu 1989). In such a process one may find a tension arises when habituated and embodied ways of experiencing one's self and person is forced into a field of opinion where one's usual orienting in the world is no longer sufficient. Living in such a tension, I suggest, may produce collective bodily pains and symptoms. One should keep in mind that Bourdieu's 'habitus' does not pertain to the dispositions of the individual only, but to the community (ibid:80). Further, Bourdieu points out that habitus is a 'universalizing mediation which causes the individual agent's practice' (ibid:79). In line with such ideas, a person is not a closed and completed entity. Rather, he or she is ready and open to connect with and enter relationships with other selves and surroundings. As such, the person may be seen as a unit that actively interprets new situations with new meanings and experiences of wholeness. Simultaneously, it gives an opportunity to analyse the tensions and pain within the individual bodies and selves, as well as the community, as moments of difficulties in the self's reorientation and changes of habits and practices.

In order to deepen the understanding of Tamil diffuse illnesses and ways of curing one step further, it seems necessary to combine and interpret the data from everyday life in Norway within a context of Hindu social and religious practice. Aspects regarding psychological and social themes of dependence/autonomy, communality/individuality and separation/fusion become of special interest. The way a person relates to such dimensions in personal and social life is highly formed by ways of upbringing, expectations and duties throughout the lifecycle and the meaning related to these practices. By looking into what may be seen as constituting significant parts of a Hindu self and a Hindu inner world, Tamil experiences in Arctic Harbor should be illuminated.

One needs to acknowledge the Hindu-Tamil self not only as a socio-centric self, but also as a kind of 'metaphysical self' (Morris 1994). It is evident that in an Indian, and I add a Hindu-Tamil context on Sri Lanka, metaphysical concepts drawn from Brahmanic traditions penetrate the wider cultural world and social practices (Morris 1994). Concepts such as moksha, dharma and karma[8] constitute what anthropologist and psychoanalyst, Sudhir Kakar (1997), has called the 'Hindu world image' that gives structure and meaning to everyday life for ordinary people. Without going into a discussion of Hindu metaphysics, I will only remark that the mentioned concepts seems to provide guidelines for living that in various ways highlight the dimensions of fusion, dependency and communality. Whether such central concepts within a Hindu-world-image are consciously acknowledged or codified in elaborate rituals, Kakar says: 'this image is so much in a Hindu's bones that he may not be aware of it' (ibid:15), but still deeply influences the way Hindus think and act. And I might add; also influence how Tamil Hindus feel, perceive and experience their life and surroundings.

Taking part in religious practice seems of great significance in Tamil everyday life and in monitoring health and sickness. As Fuller notes: 'ordinary [Hindu] people see relationships with the deities as fundamental in their lives' (Fuller 1992: 5). Generally, one may say that Hindus tend to live in a theistic universe in the sense that they believe that the gods, male and female, and also various spirits, exist (ibid.). Because they exist, the deities may also be prayed to for help and are seen as a source of hope and cure in undertaking fortunes and misfortunes as well as the activities that are essential for day-to-day living. All together, Tamils may be seen as vulnerable to the experience of not being part of a Tamil wholeness that supplies and regulates everyday social practice by principals of kin and caste as it is embedded in a Hindu context.

As in the cases presented and in my general material, Tamil refugees in Arctic Harbor may well be described as adrift and loosing hold of their regular everyday life. In this situation the often unconscious Hindu life-philosophy may emerge as implicitly significant, but with no longer appropriate or sufficient guidelines in orienting themselves in the radical new social, cultural and ecological environment, and thus producing strong existential feelings of being alone and vulnerable. By this perspective, one may see the Tamils as finding, often unconscious metaphysical ideas and motivations, crucial in experiences related to states of health and sensations of well-being. As such motivations are seen as unconscious but of significance for existential and meaningful experiences, they may be understood as habituated and thus part of an embodied knowledge. Considering this knowledge as contained in Tamil bodies, one may understand how they might be expressed through a language of the body. As significant parts of such embodied knowledge or habituated patterns no longer fit the new social, climatic and cultural world surrounding the Tamils in Arctic Harbor, it becomes possible to see the body as expressing such a misfit in ways of diffuse kinds of illnesses.

Not only does a misfit between habituated patterns regarding experiences of self and person and the radically new surroundings be ways of understanding some of the divers vague Tamil aches and pains. This perspective might also open for an understanding of what Tamils on an existential or metaphysical level are seeking when striving to restore and cure such suffering. When Tamils reconstruct bits and pieces of Ayurvedic medical approaches and other traditional practices for healing, it may not only be seen as a medical approach as such. It can also be seen as a search for a context of meaning that provides a confirmation and experience of the Tamil individual as part of social system and a metaphysical cosmology that is precarious for Tamils' sense of identity and well-being. Within such a view, one may also see that Tamil religious life and search for community supply a significant contribution within a pluralistic and flexible understanding of medical and health promoting practices, as well as self and body.

Summing up

By way of concluding, I will briefly sum up the aim and argument in this paper. The point of departure for this study refers to the many Tamils that experience diffuse and vague aches and pains that are difficult to diagnose and cure for

Norwegian health personal. When confronted with Norwegian physicians and staff that are trained in biomedicine, the Tamils are also implicitly (and unconsciously) challenged by Norwegian and Westernised views of self and personhood that separates body from soul and individual from social. Among Tamils such distinctions are not common and are rather treated as a whole, as pertains for Tamil Ayurvedic medicine and traditional healing.

In the discrepancy between the two distinct medical and everyday practices, each one provides a specific context for experiences of one's self and person, I argue that Tamils deal with confusion, uncertainty and tensions regarding identity and well-being. Additionally, since most Tamils seem to have only fragmented knowledge of traditional healing approaches and 'there is no one to ask or talk with', this may be seen to deepen a bewildering puzzlement connected to health and selfhood. Simultaneously, the reconstruction of parts and bits of Ayurvedic medicine alongside a variety of other healing practices, also tends to supply comfort, healing and confirmation of self-identity.

Opening for perspectives that see the body and self as an orienting point of being in the world, I point to Tamil creations of new social and religious practices that supply a context in which they may experience healing, well-being and value as social persons and (metaphysical) selves. The case of the birthday party provides an example of how Tamils may transgress traditional patterns for social stigma and thus create a form of healing within the realm of communitarian and social religious practices. By such perspectives, I aim to open for recognition of links between well-being, body and self that may be seen to create new contexts of meaning and practices within a flexible health promoting and medical plurality.

Notes

1. In the period between 1996–1999 I made several short visits to different fishing villages along the Arctic coast of Northern Norway where Tamils have settled. During my one to three weeks' stays, I did participant-observation and conducted interviews among the Tamil population and healthcare staff.

2. Tamils are the most numerous and stable refugee population in Northern Norway. Among the approximately eight thousand Tamils in Norway, three thousands live in the three northernmost *fylker* (counties) and about a thousand of these live in the small fishing villages of Finnmark County. For more than ten years, the Tamil population has been part of northern fishing village communities. In some of these villages the Tamil population has increased to about 10 per cent of the total population which ranges between 1500–3000 inhabitants within the villages. With only a few exceptions all Tamil men and women work in the fishing industry in menial, but well paid positions such as 'cutters' (cutting whole fish with a sharp knife).

3. In the period from 1996–1999 I conducted nine fieldwork visits in Finnmark, each between one to three weeks in duration. I employed the methods of participant-observation and conducted approximately thirty in-depth interviews. The study was funded by the Psychosocial Team for Refugees, Northern Norway and Psychiatric Research in Finnmark and Troms (PFFT).

4. September 1999 I was granted a four year scholarship by the University of Trondheim, NTNU (Norwegian University of Science and Technology).
5. Arctic Harbor is a pseudonym.
6. Finnmarksvidda is mostly inhabited by the indigenous Sami populations that traditionally make a living as reindeer (caribou) herdsmen. Along the coast there is a more mixed population consisting of Sami peoples combining fishing and reindeer keeping and non-Sami Norwegian inhabitants.
7. Arctic Harbor is one of several fishing communities along the northern coast of Norway, where there is a substantial settlement of Tamils. From a national and political perspective such communities are regarded as isolated and marginal, dependent on the whims of nature and the fishing industry. Nevertheless, the settlements are considered of great importance to the national economy and social structure (Brox 1987), which provide arguments for national subsidies to the fishing industry, the establishment of a modern infra-structure and a minimum of social welfare.
8. See for instance Kakar 1997.

References

Bauman, Z. 1995. *Modernity and Ambivalence*. Cambridge: Polity Press.

Bourdieu, P. 1989. *Outline of a Theory of Practice*. Cambridge: Cambridge University Press.

Brox, O. 1987. 'The Peripheri as "Buffer" in a Mixed Economy', *Sociology Today* 3–4: 35–45.

Buijs, G. (ed.) 1996. *Migrant Women. Crossing Boundaries and Changing Identities*. Oxford: Berg.

Csordas, T.J. 1994. *Embodiment and Experience. The Existential Ground of Culture and Self*. Cambridge: Cambridge University Press.

Daniel, V. 1997. 'Suffering Nation and Alienation', in A. Kleinman, V. Das and M. Lock. (eds) *Social Suffering*. Berkeley, California: University of California Press, 309–358.

Daniel, V. and J.C. Knudsen (eds) 1995. *Mistrusting Refugees*. Berkeley: University of California Press.

Dumont, L. 1980. *Homo Hierachicus. The Caste System and Its Implications*. Chicago: The University of Chicago.

Fuller, C.J. 1992. *The Camphor Flame. Popular Hinduism and Society in India*. Princeton: Princeton University Press.

Geertz, C. 1973. *The Interpretation of Cultures*. New York: Harper Torchbooks.

Giddens, A. 1991. *Modernity and Self-identity. Self and Society in the Late Modern Age*. Cambridge: Polity Press.

Goffman, E. 1961. *Encounters. Two Studies in the Sociology of Interaction*. Indianapolis: Boobs Merrill Educational Publishing.

Grønseth, A.S. 1997. 'Tamils Cannot Live Alone', *Lines* No. 1/7. Psychosocial Center for Refugees. Oslo: University of Oslo.

——2001. 'In Search of Community: A Quest for Wellbeing among Tamil Refugees in Northern Norway', *Medical Anthropology Quarterly* 15(4): 493–514.

Hahn, R. 1984. 'Rethinking 'Illness' and "Disease"', in V. Daniel and J. Pugh (eds) *Contributions to Asian Studies. Vol. 18, South Asian systems of Healing*, Leiden: E. J. Brill, 1–23.

Jackson, M. 1989. *Paths toward a Clearing: Radical Empiricism and Ethnographic Inquiry*. Bloomington: Indiana University Press.

Jacobson-Widding, A. and D. Westerlund (eds) 1989. *Culture, Experience and Pluralism. Essays on African Ideas of Illness and Healing*. Upsala: Acta Univesitatis Upsaliensis. Uppsala Studies in Cultural Anthropology-13.

Jenkins, J. 1996. 'The Impress of Extremity: Women's Experience of Trauma and Political Violence', in C. Sargent and C. Brettell (eds) *Gender and Health. An International Perspective*. New Jersey: Prentice-Hall, 278–291.

Kakar, S. 1997 [1978]. *The Inner World. A Psychoanalytic Study of Childhood and Society in India*. Oxford: Oxford University Press.

Kleinman, A. 1980. *Patients and Healers in the Context of Culture. An Exploration of the Borderland between Anthropology, Medicine, and Psychiatry*. Berkeley: University of California Press.

Loudon, J.B. (ed.) 1976. *Social Anthropology and Medicine*. London: Academic Press.

Lutz, C. 1988. *Unnatural Emotions. Everyday Sentiments on a Micronesian Atoll and their Challenge to Western Theory*. Chicago: Chicago University Press.

Marriot, M. 1976. 'Hindu Transactions: Diversity Without Dualism', in B. Kapferer (ed.) *Transaction and Meaning: Directions in the Anthropology of Exchange and Symbolic Behaviour*. Philadelphia: Institute for the Study of Human Issues, 109–142.

Merleau-Ponty, M. 2002 [1945]. *Phenomenology of Perception*. London: Routledge.

Mines, M. 1988. 'Conceptualizing the Person: Hierarchical Society and Individual Autonomy in India', *American Anthropologist* 90: 568–579.

Morris, B. 1994. *Anthropology of the Self. The Individual in Cultural Perspective*. London: Pluto Press.

Rosaldo, M. 1980. *Knowledge and Passion: Ilongot Notions of Self and Social life*. Cambridge: Cambridge University Press.

Samson, C. (ed.) 1999. *Health Studies. A Critical and Cross-Cultural Reader*. Oxford: Blackwell Publishers.

11

The War of the Spiders

Constructing Mental Illnesses in the
Multicultural Communities of the
Highlands of Chiapas

Witold Jacorzynski

How do contemporary Maya Indians from Chiapas satisfy their medical needs in new, multicultural, heterogeneous, highly stratified and conflicting communities? How do they negotiate between national, and 'modern' medical systems, and local, traditional systems? This chapter proposes to answer these questions using as a case study the experience of Trifena, a Tzotzil woman suffering from schizophrenia and epilepsy.

Our case study is multifaceted and emerges as a result of interference of three dimensions: the medical systems in a globalised and pluricultural world, the ethnic and social situation of the living Maya Indian groups in the Highlands of Chiapas and, so-called mental illnesses as they appear and as they are interpreted and treated in the region. The anthropological literature emphasised one or two of the aforementioned aspects, but rarely the three of them at the same time. Some authors try to describe the core of the pluriethnic and globalised medicines (Janzen 1978, Kleinmann 1980, Lupton 1994, Nichter and Nichter 1996), others have written on the specific topics related to indigenous medicine in the Highlands of Chiapas envisaged as a dynamic, syncretic system (Holland 1963, Köhler 1974, 1995, Beltran 1986). Very few tried to analyse the pluricultural indian medicines situating the healing process in the postmodern, pluricultural and globalised context of the Chiapas region (Ayora Díaz 1998, Freyermuth 2000). I will follow those authors while at the same time avoiding their highly macro/etic-oriented inclination.

In this chapter I propose to focus on the ideas that have been expressed by Kleinman (1980, 1995) and Good (1994) although many of them have always been present in most interpretative mainstreams of anthropology in the twentieth century.

The first and foremost goal of medical anthropology is an interpretation of the interpretations. Kleinman says that 'a central concern in ethnography should be the interpretation of what is at stake for particular participants in particular situations. That orientation will lead the ethnographer to collective (both local and societal) and individual (both public and intimate) levels of analysis of experience-near interests that, we hold, offer a more valid initial understanding of what are social-psychological characteristics of forms of life in local worlds than either professional sociological categories (roles, sets, status) or psychological terminology (affect, cognition, defense, behaviour)' (Kleinman 1995: 98).

The expression of 'what is at stake' must be understood in reference to the social experience of both individuals and an ethnographer. On the one side 'experience may, on theoretical grounds, be thought of as the intersubjective medium of social transactions in local moral worlds' (Kleinman 1995: 97), with such characteristics as existential pressure for coherence and unity, the immediacy of its felt quality and the confusing multiplicity and indeterminancy of its flow (Kleinman 1995: 99). The ethnographer must enter the social experience at a particular time and place and match 'how individuals encounter the flow of experience'. Individuals do not invent it, they are 'borne or thrown into the stream of lived interactions' (Kleinman 1995: 98).

Experience of the individuals gives origin to the 'explanatory models' of individuals involved in a healing situation, including the ethnographer: 'Explanatory models are their notions about an episode of sickness and its treatment that are employed by all those engaged in the clinical process' (Kleinman 1980: 105). The explanatory models originate in the belief-systems or, to use the Wittgensteinian word, a *Weltbild*.

The explanatory models need to be contextualised in the aforementioned experience and can be analysed from the point of view of the meta-explanatory model construed by the anthropologist. This meta-model should correspond roughly to what Wittgenstein called *übersichtliche Darstellung*, a perspicuous representation that 'describes our form of presentation, the way we see things' (Wittgenstein 1985: 24). The perspicuous representations differ from discipline to discipline and from perspective to perspective but one thing is clear: it gives a 'Gestalt' to our data, it shapes its 'Gesicht', its 'Physiognomie' (Schulte 2001: 111).

I will assume for the sake of discussion that certain metaphors and allegories constitute the perspicuous representation of the ethnographical material and therefore possess a 'surplus meaning', give us knowledge or comprehension of 'what is at stake'. This point of view was emphasised in different contexts by philosophers (Black 1962, Ricoeur 1979, Lakoff and Johnson 1980) and anthropologists (Clifford 1986: 98). In the last paragraph I will try to use a metaphor of William Blake to give a 'surpluss meaning' to the story of Trifena. Now, its high time we start to describe the social experience of different actors and their explanatory models.

My first encounters with Trifena

I met Trifena in December 1998, when she was visiting her brother Samuel in Chibtik, her native community situated in a township Chenalho' in the Highlands of Chiapas. I went to live in Samuel and his wife Martha's house with the purpose of collecting data about Samuel's Pacinsa lineage and its role in the introduction of the Presbyterian Church in Chibtik in the early 1950s. Manuel and his brother Victorio were two 'religious heroes' who struggled together in the early 1950s to create a new community, Chibtik, and adopted Presbyterianism. The fight ended successfully. The lineage of Pacinsa succeeded in creating a new community on the periphery of Xunuch, the bigger community reigned by other lineages. Thanks to Victorio and Manuel, the Pacinsa emerged as a new ruling lineage in a new place.

I wanted to use Trifena's narrative as additional material, which could throw light on the religious conflicts in the area, but finally I realised that her story had a life of its own. She was desperately looking for somebody to speak Spanish with. Most of the inhabitants of the village are monolingual, Tzotzil-speaking Maya Indians. Trifena told me that she forgot Tzotzil while she lived for the last ten years on the island Cozumel located on the Yucatan coast, a place well known for its tourist charms. Her appearance testified to what she said: she wore shorts and a t-shirt, clothes used by mestizo women from the Caribbean coast but not by conservative, traditionally dressed Tzotzil women from the township of Chenalho'. After I spoke to her various times I realised that she was forced to come back from Cozumel because of her illness and because she had commited 'adultery'. Although she did not mention this part of the story, her brother did it for her. He told me that it was he who brought her back after he met her up in Cozumel where he was working as a seasonal construction worker. Two or three Indian families from Chibtik emigrated to Cozumel and helped their relatives from Chiapas to find a job. Samuel and Trifena's sister Benita married a Maya Indian from Yucatan and found a job in a supermarket. She invited Samuel to stay with her and her husband. It was then, in December 1998, that he met Trifena, in a 'pitiful condition'. She had just been abandoned by her husband Daniel, a man born in the same village, to whom she had given two children. Samuel mentioned two reasons for the collapse of her marriage: one was that, as her husband maintained, she committed adultery with José, his younger brother, and the other, that, as Samuel suggested, she became very ill with *chuvaj* and *tup'-ik'* and became an unbearable burden to her husband. *Tup'-ik'* means in Tzotzil to 'cut out a breath' and corresponds roughly to epilepsy syndrome while *chuvaj* can be translated as madness.

When I visited Chibtik the next month, Trifena no longer lived with Samuel's family but in her father's hut. I visited her there and was a witness of one of her attacks. One day when Don Manuel, her father and I were drinking *pozol*, a cold maize beverage, she suddenly turned her head and started mumbling incomprehensible words in a low voice, her eyes bugged out like a frog, and her body started moving uncontrollably. After five minutes or so she was alert again and she told us she did not remember anything. What she is conscious of is that *xkopojik te ta sjol*, they talk in her head. She reported that one voice on the right side of her chest says 'PU' and the other, on the left side of her chest, speaks out 'JE'. She identifies PU with *Pukuj*, which in Tzotzil means Demon, evil, and *JE* with Jesus. Don Manuel told me that sometimes she becomes violent, starts running somewhere, runs away to the forest, climbs the mountains, gives sermons on the Last Judgment to everybody, falls down on the ground, grinds her teeth, and spits out a lot of foam. Violent, unsociable and uncontrollable action was an example of *chuvaj* while epilepsy-like attacks were a manifestation of *tup'-ik'*.

'Why do they talk to me? What do they want?' Trifena asked me when I was about to leave Don Manuel's place. I said nothing.

Ali Kajvaltik spas preba: the God makes a test

Within the next few months Trifena moved out of her father's house and started living in her brother Eliseo's hut. I realised that she was a burden to everybody. She had no money, no job; she inspired fear in children when she suffered from the attacks. Her father and Samuel reacted with violence. They tied her to the bed or to the wooden pole supporting the hut construction. Sometimes she screamed, groaned, urinated where she was tied. As she told me:

> When my brother Samuel brought me here to Chibtik, my illness got worse. I used to set off running, I talked to myself, I escaped at nights to the mountains. My brother used to tie me up when I used to picked up a stick to hit them, they could not catch me. Once they tied me up and they closed me in a hut alone. And I was there talking and screaming and many came to watch me...

Trifena's Presbyterian family, which includes her brothers Eliseo and Samuel as well as her father Don Manuel, from the beginning imposed on her their own interpretation of her illness. Don Manuel told me in 1999:

> It is a demon who gave this illness, this is why Trifena is ill. The Demon tests us, whether we have obeyed the word of God, he sends us the illness. But God wants our hearts not to be discouraged; He wants us to pay attention to God's Word.

When I asked him who exactly sends us an illness, God or the Demon, he said: 'The Demon gives us an illness, the God does not. Let us ask our heads and hearts to be strong. Let us obey God'. When I mentioned that Trifena heard Jesus and the Demon talking in her head, he nodded:

When she speaks with someone who seems to be God, she hears somebody talking. But this is a message from the Demon alone. Who really speaks a lot to her is the Demon.

If it is the Demon who tries to play God in Trifena's head, when does she access to God's real Word? This is the question a religious man in Chibtik answers in the same way. One can listen to God's Word in the temple, following the rules officially established by the spiritual Presbyterian authorities. The other Presbyterian members of the Pacinsa lineage followed the interpretation of Don Manuel. They agree that the *pukuj ioch ta yo'onton Trifena* (the Demon penetrated into the heart of Trifena) because God tests her faith. When I asked them whether Trifena's faith had to do with the supposed adultery she had committed in Cozumel they defended their sister and admitted that she had not committed any sin. As Samuel put it:

It did not come from the depth of her heart that she committed sin with another man, it was because she was ill.

Eliseo added to it:

I think this is the work of the Demon, the illness exists only when we are on the earth. The savior is Jesus.

But Marta, wife of Samuel and a daughter of the present pastor of Chibtik, Pedro Xupun, who belongs to the same lineage as Daniel, Trifena's husband, suggests that Trifena contracted her illness as a punishment for her adultery: 'She committed sin with another man'.

As a remedy to the *chuvaj* and *tup'-ik'* the Presbyterians recommended prayers to God, attendance to the temple and herbs given to people by God.

A traditional medicine-woman Micaela: 'This is something precious which she did not know how to appreciate'

Micaela is the wife of Elías, a first cousin of Trifena, Samuel, Eliseo and Juan. As a little boy Elías emigrated to San Cristóbal in search of work and education. After years of suffering and mistreatment from mestizo *patrones* he finished secondary school and university supported by a scholarship from the Mexican Government. He decided to stay in San Cristóbal rather than to go back to Chibtik. In San Cristóbal he married Micaela, a teacher from Candelaria, a traditional Indian community located in Chamula township. Although Elías came from a Presbyterian family he recognised the traditional knowledge of his wife, who in her youth had received a spiritual gift from God to cure people. In 1999 Elías, who lived in San Cristóbal, and at that time was my student, told me that Trifena went to his wife Micaela, under the supervision of her oldest brother Juan. Elías witnessed a ceremony set up in Micaela's and his house:

> I felt that my head stood on end. My wife saw with her eyes that something like a buzzard flew out. My older brothers, the mestizo doctors, cannot help Trifena because they do not know anything about the soul's illnesses. If she chooses to do evil, if she chooses to do the Demon's work, she can turn into a very powerful and dangerous woman. She can provide help as well as send illnesses to women and men of the world. If she accepts what is good, she will only have little power to help other women and men.

Elías, in his endeavour to interpret Trifena followed Micaela: 'She was a real master of ceremonies and she took a risk to deal with the Demon and God in Trifena's body'. She was willing to carry out two other ceremonies. During the second one she would give to the Demon candles and *pox* (Maya alcoholic beverage made of sugar cane) so that he could leave Trifena's body. In the third ceremony, Trifena had to accept her mission from God and turn into a medicine-woman. But Trifena and Juan never came back. In 2000 I was able to interview Micaela about her impression of Trifena's illness. She explained to me that Trifena must die if she does not want to obey God. Traditional Maya Indians believe that God reveals his will to man or woman in what apparently looks like *tup'-ik'* and in dreams. The problem she sees is that Trifena's family, which is also Elías's family, lacks religiousness and does not give her any spiritual support. Many months after the ceremony, Micaela saw Trifena in Juan's house and, as she reported to me, she gave her some advice:

> 'That's it', I tell her, 'it will talk for your whole life long. If you do not have faith and do not cope with it... You will always hear it but if you try to get better, you will see, there is a solution because what you had, what you have, isn't it something which you were about to receive, something beautiful?! But because your family does not know about this and they do not believe, what happened is that you lost it, you lost it because of what you did.'

I asked Micaela how it was that a Demon had entered her body and how one can know whether she or he has an ordinary *tup'-ik'* or a message from God. She explained to me that she saw in her dream that Trifena fell down in a pit in Cozumel and got possessed by the soul of an unidentified dead man. As for God's message, Micaela can, as many other medicine-women from the Highlands of Chiapas, diagnose illnesses by checking the pulse of the patient. This way, they believe, they get knowledge about the state of the *sch'ulel* (the soul), which lives in the blood and heart of all living beings.

A modern neurosurgeon Dr Araujo:
'This is an illness like any other'

After Trifena spent a year in the hut of her father and another year with the family of Eliseo, her brother, she travelled to San Cristóbal and came to live with Juan, her older brother. It was amazing for me to imagine that the oldest son of Don Manuel, a Presbyterian as well, could take his sister to a traditional medicine-woman. When I finally met him personally in 2000, the spell did not break. Juan was a charming person with a lot of theories about Trifena's illness, a 'scientifically' oriented man, a pragmatist, a hybrid personality. He was proud of studying at a local university for Indian teachers and about to receive a Bachelor's Degree in Education. He confessed to me that because he had been 'scientifically' investigating his sister's illness, he had to try as many hypotheses as possible. A visit to Micaela, a traditional Tzotzil witch, was only one among many experiments he was considering to help his sister. He also tried, among others, *vomoletik*, medicinal plants; Presbyterian prayers; a traditional soup made of humming birds; toad's substance, reported in one of the illustrated magazines as a means to cure schizophrenia in Australia; injecting vitamins; and a therapeutic system of breathing. When I suggested to him that we could try modern medicine, he did not hesitate.

In the course of 2000 and 2001 we travelled three times to Tuxtla Gutierrez, the capital of the state of Chiapas in order to consult a neurosurgeon Dr Araujo, from a private clinic. During the first visit, without any interview, the doctor made preliminary clinical tests 'in order to exclude an organic tumor' and admitted that Trifena had developed epilepsy lobuli temporal, a 'totally organic' disease, treatable with pharmacological measures. He prescribed drugs, epamin and mysolin, and told the patient to take the medication fifteen minutes before breakfast, lunch and dinner. He also gave Juan a booklet on the curing of epileptic patients and asked him to note the time and circumstances of the possible epileptic attacks. After the first visit the voices in Trifena's head stopped, she got fat and nervously alert. During the second visit, he told Juan to administer a stronger dose of the same medication. During the third visit, after Trifena's family realised that the voices had started again, he defended the diagnosis:

> There are many causes of why the attacks occur, many causes which facilitate the occurrence of the attacks. The brain, the neurons, they have learned to convulse. They do nothing but look for any excuse. Those neurons which are badly educated, will be re-educated by us.

When I asked him about the voices she hears he said:

> Unfortunately, there are psychiatric symptoms as well, aren't there; that they hear things, that they see things, that the voices tell them not to do something, or they want to kill them, or they persecute them. But this is a hallucination. The

nightmares are very frequent symptoms. A symptom taken seriously by people, is what has been seen, what has been lived through.

Dr Araujo and Trifena then had the following dialogue:

Dr Araujo: 'And you have had your nightmares?'
Trifena: 'Yes'
Dr Araujo: 'What were your nightmares?'
Trifena: 'What? I truly do not remember, I was hearing voices.'
Dr Araujo: 'What did they tell you? Did they insult you, did they threaten you, did they call you?'
Trifena: 'What I heard was just: "I am God" or whatever, only the pure names of Satan were said. That is why I think, I thought that it is Satan who was talking in my head.'
Dr Araujo: 'Satan does not exist! Satan does not exist! Does he? He exists only for those who believe in him. You are cured at the moment in which you do not have any symptoms. At this moment you are cured. But you have to keep on taking drugs.'

Juan asked the neurosurgeon if the traditional means of curing like prayers and herbs interfere with the scientific ones. Doctor Araujo replied:

There are people who dedicate themselves to exploiting other people. They say they can cure you with this. The herbs are good, you see. The drugs are extracted from the herbs, but with a technique, with knowledge... No, there is no miraculous medication...

While Juan was repeating 'there is no...', the neurosurgeon went on saying that neither the Virgin, nor witchcraft, nor dogs which she came across, nor the Moon has anything to do with what Trifena suffers. What she has is but simple post-traumatic epilepsy originated in 'damaged neurons'. As a cure he prescribed more mysolin 1–1–1 instead of 1–1/2–1/2 explaining that:

O.K. I will increase the dosage. Take, for example a sweater for cold. With a thin sweater, I feel better, but I still feel cold. Good, I will give you a bigger sweater, and I felt the cold less. But still you feel cold. So I will give you a sweater and a coat. I am fine with this. Good, this is what I need for her.

Trifena: the interludium

After a third visit to Dr Araujo in 2001 Trifena came to live with Juan and his wife Priscilla in San Cristóbal. Although the dosage of epamin was increased, and we cooperated to buy the drugs, Trifena was not doing well. She used either to forget to take the drug or it was not supplied on time. The voices were talking again but this time they multiplied and moved to the throat: She heard the voice of Daniel, her husband, San Juan, the Baptist, the Holy Spirit, Peter and Paul the apostles. When she visited me in September 2001 in my office located in CIESAS, the Center for Advanced Studies and Research in Social Anthropology located on the outskirts of San Cristóbal she was all shaken. She gave me the drawing, which she had made for me two weeks before, entitled *ja' vu'un* (this is me). 'Whom did you draw here?', I asked her. Trifena points to a drawing of a girl and reads what she wrote below the picture: 'They are talking in my body. I hear voices: they say that it is Jesus'. Our dialogue continued:

Witold: 'You are smiling...'
Trifena: 'No, I am just like that. In my body they are talking. I feel it in my head. The voice, which is in the middle of the throat, is the Holy Spirit. It talks well to me. Different words. It says: "I am your God". Another voice speaks to me in the right part of my head. Some time ago, it spoke badly. Bad words sometimes. In the middle of the head. I felt that it spoke to me. That it enters.'

Trifena touches her throat several times. Then she continues: 'This time it entered my throat. It is the Holy Spirit. He speaks well to me: "your child... who takes care of them? Where are they? Do you love Daniel?" He asked me that. I do not answer. I have not spoken to Daniel for two years. "Daniel loves you. Do not see another man. You have to wait for him. You are married. You have to wait for him". This is what he says: "I am the Holy Spirit". He is talking right now: "I am your Holy Spirit"'.

Trifena touches her throat again. She mentions other voices as she hears them: a voice telling her about her children and telling her to visit them. One voice negates what the other says: 'It is not true', it says, 'it is not true'. Then again, the voice of the Holy Spirit: 'The proof of faith, and the proof of love. It's proof of faith is about whether I have faith in God and the proof of love is about whether you love Daniel...'. This voice is again interrupted by the voice of Satan: 'She is faithful but it is not true. It is faith of love, but of Satan. It's good that she knows Spanish...'

At that moment the voice of the Holy Spirit told her that the other voice, which spoke to her, was the voice of Satan. Then she calmed down. After a while she told me that at night she had heard another voice in her throat. This time it was the voice of the apostles Peter and Paul. They had spoken to her about her children. She had cried. The dialogues of the voices she hears are not only polarised and conflicting, they are also bilingual. The bad voice speaks to her in Tzotzil and the Holy Spirit talks to her in Spanish. But then they change. Trifena is exhausted. I am depressed. I give her money for her drawings. She disappears.

Juan: *My mind is absurd, isn't it?*

From this time on, Trifena moved constantly: she lived with Juan, with the family of her uncle in San Cristóbal, in the house of her sister in San Cristóbal (see Table 11.1). Juan was worried. Although sometimes he overreacted and used to beat her with a stick, he was always ready to help and work out new solutions. In 2002 I started convincing him to undertake a new shock therapy. I insisted that Trifena must go back to Cozumel, have a talk with Daniel, accept the truth whatever it means, see her children. Juan agreed. I paid for their bus tickets and we were ready to go. Trifena was happy. She told me that she would be willing to stay longer in Cozumel if this were the wish of her husband. Juan explained to me that the journey would help her to free her mind and take everything off her chest. On the other hand he was ready to corroborate 'scientifically' another hypothesis he had worked out: Trifena's soul was lost in the ocean and when she recuperated it with prayers, she would be cured. When we reached the shores of Cozumel after seventeen hours travel by bus and one hour by ferry, Trifena was overswept by strong emotions. We met her friends, people from the Presbyterian Church she had once known and loved and finally arrived at Benita's place. A small, poor hut made of sticks with a big television set and a toaster inside it. Benita had a job. She had managed to get a job in a mall. Then we visited Trifena's husband Daniel and the children. Daniel was gloomy when he saw us but he made himself get up and shook our hands. He said coldly *hola* to Trifena while she was trying to stand aside and to talk with her children. They were timid but received her well. In a few minutes she embraced them. Ricardo, her older son, was twelve and Gerardo was six. Juan arranged a meeting with Daniel. Trifena asked him if she could take the children for a walk. He agreed and we went off to wander around the city of Cozumel and on the seashore. I saw Juan entering the sea and asking the sea to free his sister's soul. In the evening Trifena, Juan and I went to the medicine-woman's house to exorcise Trifena. The children stayed in Benita's house playing with Benita's child.

The medicine-woman, called Sister Alicia, belonged to the Pentecostal Church and was a friend of Benita. She explained to us that Satan, who had violated her one night, entering her womb, possessed Trifena's body. Although Trifena did not remember anything, the medicine-woman and her husband started the ceremony. They tried to pull Satan out of Trifena's body. *'Fuera Satanás, fuera'* (Out, Out Satan), they cried and sobbed and yelled. Trifena was spitting out a lot of phlegm and was writhing and yelling too.

After the ceremony we went back to Benita's house to meet Daniel. He was waiting for us. There were three families around and Daniel's friends who wanted to listen to the speeches. I approached with a taperecorder. Daniel looked upset but he did not say a word. Juan was the oldest son of Don Manuel, a spiritual leader of the Presbyterian Church and he was a master of ceremonies. Daniel respected him, whatever happened. After a long introductory speech by Juan, Daniel was interrogated in Tzotzil. Juan wanted him to confess why he had abandoned his wife and how it came about that she got ill. He wanted to know as well if Daniel would accept her again. Daniel told us that Trifena had seen the letters 'P U' in a church while they were listening to *Palabra de Dios*, God's word. He took Trifena several times to a doctor. He remembered that the doctor gave her pills for parasites, but he could not remember what the name of the illness was. '*Tup'-ik*', Epilepsy', said Juan. 'Yes, mental epilepsy', added Daniel. He argued, however, that it was not because of her illness that they separated. It was because Trifena committed a *smul*, a sin. He started complaining about what had happened three years before:

> But when she does not give you anything to eat, if she takes care of your younger or older brother, if she gives food to him, washes his clothes, but does not take care of you; you think this is all right? Sometimes I am hungry when I get home at noon, she does not give me anything to eat. One time I got back home to eat, she did not respect me. 'Go and bring some eggs to prepare them', I said to one of my children. He was still little and I had to take money from her, because it is she who keeps money. I gave money to him, but she stole the money back from the little one, and I did not eat anything. If we tell everything about what happened it will never end. This is what they did with my younger brother: they waited till I sleep, you understand, we live together in the same house, he is not separated [my brother], they wait until I sleep. As it is in this case, they put more water on the beans, they go to sleep at eleven, twelve, while I sleep at ten, half past ten. Her heart was ready to do what they did to me.

Juan insisted that Trifena must ask Daniel again to forgive her. But he knew well it would not change anything. Daniel was positive about that. As he put it:

> She said to me: 'Forgive me, I will come back to you'. 'This cannot be', I told her. This is what I did... you asked me a lot. In this way, I did it from the beginning, because I knew it, I talked with God, I only did what had to be done... only this.

After Juan realised that Daniel would not forgive Trifena, he asked her to speak. He asked her what 'love' and 'respect' for her husband were. We waited in silence to hear Trifena's answer but she did not say a word. After the interrogation was finished, Daniel took the children and was about to switch on the engine of his motorbike, when Trifena approached them. They talked for a while. Then Daniel and the children disappeared in the darkness. Trifena told us that she asked him to let her spend the night with the children in Benita's house but the small ones preferred to go to *feria*. But they promised to come back the next morning. Trifena was sad. I saw her entering Benita's house and heard her crying and telling her sister that it was not true what her husband said. I was tired and went to sleep in a hammock. The stars and the moon were rising. Suddenly, somebody touched me. I heard someone sobbing. It was Trifena.

> You brought me here, Don Victor... but I would not have come, I would not have
> seen my children, I would not have remembered anything... you brought me
> here... it would have been better if I had not come.

I felt strange. Guilty? Was I guilty? I unwrapped myself from the hammock.
We went off to take a walk.

> You have to confront it; you have to ask him for a divorce. He must give you
> money to live on, he must let you see your children.

I felt she understood. Next morning Trifena was waiting for her children but
they did not show up. We went to the medicine-woman to finish the
exorcism. Sister Alicia and her husband tried again to pull the Demon out of
Trifena's body. 'Out, Out Satan' they cried and sobbed and yelled. Trifena
was spitting out a lot of phlegm and was writhing and yelling too. Juan who
witnessed the whole scene, whispered to me: 'I wanted to take the phlegm to
the laboratory. My mind is absurd, isn't it?'
  I remained silent.
  On our way back San Cristóbal, the three of us planned a divorce, which
was supposed to bring Trifena money and half of her house. I offered my help
in finding a good lawyer. When we parted in San Cristóbal, I thought I had
done my duty. Trifena's life was about to change.
  For a few days Trifena was feeling very well. She was planning her new life.
But when I saw her a week after our return from Cozumel, the voices were
talking again. She told me that Daniel's voice was telling her to wait for him.

> Witold: 'Don't you remember what Daniel told you in Cozumel?'
> Trifena: 'No, I do not'
> Witold: 'He told you that he did not want to have anything to do with you'
> Trifena: 'He really told me that? I do not remember anything Don Victor, I do
> not remember.'

Juan did not loose his memory, as Trifena did, he changed his mind. He told
me that it would be impossible, for the time being, to obtain a divorce because
people from the Presbyterian Church dominated by the lineage Xupun must
first sit together with the lineage of the Pacinsa and talk. 'When will they
talk?', I asked. '*Quién sabe*' (who knows), he answered.

A spiders' war: a 'perspicuous' annotation to Trifena's story

In this case I want to focus on three themes: The pluralistic/globalised health
system in the southeastern part of Mexico as shaping and reshaping social
experience of the persons involved; the cultural confusions and
misunderstandings as one of the secondary side-effects of the process of
cross-checking different explanatory models and interpreting 'what is at

stake'; and finally the general, conspicuous comprehension of the existential situation of Trifena's case.

What stands out in the description of my encounters with Trifena and different people from the lineage Pacinsa is, on the one hand, the evolution of her own autoreflexion through the drawings she did for me; and on the other, the role of the cultural confusions and misunderstandings. To understand the varieties of her experiences, most of them forced upon her by the circumstances of life, let us consider Table 11.1 overleaf.

Trifena and the members of her lineage live in a pluricultural, globalised, mosaic-like and travel-oriented society (Agenda Estadistica Chiapas 1996: 166, Ayora Díaz 1998, Rivera 2003). The map in Figure 11.1 presents the southeastern part of Mexico where our story takes place. The ethnic mosaic of Chiapas can be appreciated from the map in Figure 11.2. Migrations, international contacts and ever-changing life situations are their everyday-life reality.[1]

Trifena's case is even more exacerbated by her illness and personal tragedy. In the last four years she has changed her place, language and customs several times. In Table 11.1, I have marked with Roman numerals the most important milestones in her life.[2] First she lives in Chibtik where she shares a Tzotzil/Presbyterian form of life, and then she moves to San Cristóbal where she adapts to the mestizo form of life of the region. After she migrates to Cozumel she must form her Tzotzil/Presbyterian family in quite new circumstances: she has mestizo friends from Cozumel who exchange ideas with her about family patterns. After she becomes ill her life changes: she loses her home. From that time on, others, mostly her lineage members decide where, with whom and how long she must stay. From 1989 until 2003 she moves place at least thirteen times. In each period she undergoes another kind of therapy and listens to different interpretations about her illness and existential situation. The explanatory models proliferate. While she lives with her father, Samuel and Eliseo, she mostly prays. Juan experiments with many therapies, which I call the mixed ones for they are strongly individualist and vary from prayers, to breathing systems, homoeopathy, exorcisms, pharmacological treatment and different religious rituals practiced by the members of at least three groups (Presbyterianism, Pentecostalism and traditional Maya religion). While living with her other brothers, the Presbyterians who believe not only in prayers but also in herbs and pharmacological medicine given to them by God, she accepts the help of an ethnographer who arranges medical consultation with a neurosurgeon from Tuxtla Gutierrez. In Cozumel she goes to a Pentecostal medicine-woman. While she lives with her, she participates in the cults of her sect *Alas de Águila* or renovated Presbyterianism.

In every place she lives she adapts herself to the conditions and explanatory models prevailing. The result of this process is her own unbalanced attitude towards her illness, the inabililty to work out a coherent explanatory model of her illness. Her experience is 'thrown' into the social

Table 11.1 *Case Trifena: most important migrations, stayings and therapies*

Year	Month	Place	Family	Kinship	Therapy
1970	?	Chibtik	Manuel/Teresa	Parents	—
1987	*Trifena emigrates to San Cristóbal to continue to attend her sixth year of primary school (I)*				
1987	?	San Cristóbal	Juan Pérez Arias	Brother	—
1989	*Trifena emigrates with Daniel to Cozumel, state Quintana Roo (II)*				
1989	?	Cozumel	Daniel Xupun	Husband	Anti-parasitic pharmacological therapy
1997	*Trifena 'commits adultery' in Cozumel and leaves her house (III)*				
1998	July	Cozumel	Benita	Sister	Exorcisms Pentecostal spiritism
1998	*Trifena gets back to Chiapas in company of her brother Samuel (IV)*				
1998	December	Chibtik	Samuel/Marta	Brother/ sister-in-law	Prayers
1999	January	Chibtik	Manuel/Maruch	Father/ step-mother	Prayers, herbs
1999	May	S.C. Col. Palestina	Juan/Priscilla	Brother/ sister-in-law	Prayers, pharmacological therapy, herbs, traditional Maya rituals
2000	May	Chibtik	Eliseo/Carmela	Brother/ sister-in-law	Pharmacological therapy, herbs, prayers
2001	May	S.C. Col. Palestina	Juan	Brother	Mixed therapies
2001	August	S.C. Col. Palestina	Hermas	Sister	Prayers
2001	October	S.C. Palestina	Juan	Brother	Mixed therapies
2002	February	S.C. Col. Morelos	Miguel Perez Gutierrez	Uncle	Prayers
2002	April	S.C. Col. Palestina	Juan	Brother	Mixed therapy
2002	May	Travel to Cozumel	Benita/William	Sister/ brother-in-law	Exorcisms Pentecostal spiritism
2002	May	S.C. Col. Palestina	Juan	Brother	Mixed medicine
2003	February	Chibtik	Manuel/ Maruch	Father/ step-mother	Prayers/herbs
2003	March	Chibtik	—	—	Mixed therapy

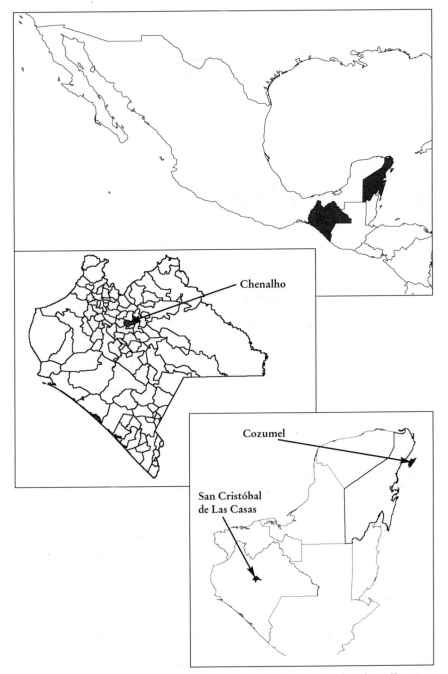

Figure 11.1 *Map showing the places where Trifena stayed, Chenalho, San Cristóbal, Cozumel*

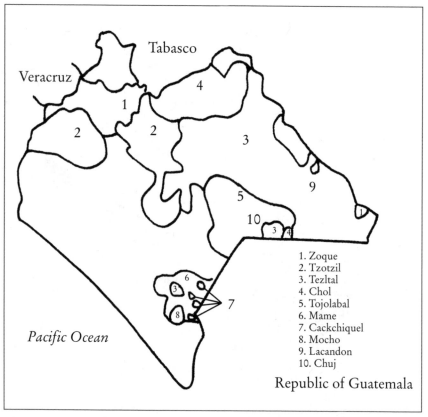

Figure 11.2 *Distribution of Indian Languages in Chiapas*

experience of the others and dominated by them. In the beginning, under the influence of Micaela, a traditional Maya healer, she believes in the original duality of her messages from the supernatural forces: On the one hand it is God who speaks to her, on the other it is Satan. But later on, the Protestant interpretation takes precedence: God's voice, and other 'good' voices she hears in the course of the development of her illness are the cover up of a demon's discourse. In the last of her drawings, when the ethnographer asks her to draw those who talk in her head, she gives him back a blank paper explaining that to make pictures of Satan is a mortal sin. The voices who lead a dialogue at first, later on become one, unidentified stream of cries and whispers. Any mission from God is excluded. She must neither speak with the voices nor understand them. The only way to survive is to pray and wait. She is, nevertheless helped in this endeavour. She finally gets separated from the family who is terrified of her attacks, interpreted as a Devil's intervention. From February 2003 she lives alone and stigmatised in an empty house in Chibtik, rarely visited by anyone.

Why is the new global pluricultural situation damaging to Trifena's well-being? I will quote only two examples of confusions and misunderstandings from which she suffered in the course of her life. The first throws light on why the pharmacological, modern medical explanatory model turned out to be useless and oppressive. First of all, the Doctor from Tuxtla Gutierrez did not do a general interview about his patient's cultural and social conditions, acting instead on the basis of his most vulgar prejudices: he prejudges that his Tzotzil patients believe in the Moon, the Virgin, witches. He prejudges that they have no knowledge of medicinal plants for as he put it *the drugs are extracted from the herbs, but with a technique, with knowledge*. For him the Maya Indians lack knowledge and therefore they fall prey to the traditional healers who 'exploit' them. He prejudges that *Satan does not exist* and that Trifena's impressions are the figment of the make-believe world of her hallucinations. He prejudges that the only way to cure her is to erase the organic symptoms she suffers. He prejudges that her illness is originated in the organic matter of the brain and must be cured only with drugs. He, finally, prejudges that the Tzotzil peasants can easily observe a discipline of drug-taking according to an exact mestizo schedule. He is condescending while using his didactic metaphors. He miscomprehends the Tzotzil culture for most of his prejudices turn out to be false. To mention only a few of them: Trifena's family does not believe in the Virgin; instead, her relatives firmly believe in the existence of Satan; they do not have three meals a day like the mestizo people from the urban environment, etc.

The other confusion takes place in Cozumel and it is Trifena who falls prey to it. Daniel refers to her failure in his dialogue with Juan. Perhaps the Tzotzil text is more relevant to understand the speaker's intentions:

Jech chak k'ucha'al lajspasik xchi'uk kitz'in xtok ne: smalaik chivay ne, ja' chava'i, ti nakalunkutik ta jun na' ne, muyuk parte ne, smalaik chivay ne.

(This is how they did with my younger brother: they wait till I sleep, you understand, we live together in the same house, he is not separated {my brother}, they wait until I sleep).

There would be nothing interesting in this passage if it were not for the strange comment by Daniel that they lived in one house. The Tzotzil word *nakalunkutik* comes from an adjective *nakal*, dwelling, residing; *kutik* is the first person exclusive plural (Laughlin 1975: 25, 247). *Nakalunkutik* can be translated as 'we (but not you) live, dwell together'. The word *chava'i* is the second person singular of *a'i*, a transitive verb which means hear, feel, understand (Laughlin 1975: 37). Using this verb, Daniel wants to emphasise that Juan must understand something, which is important and easy to overlook: Daniel, Trifena, his wife and Daniel's younger brother lived together in the same house. Trifena must have felt temptation to feel that her brother-in-law was part of her family. This situation is not accepted in

Chibtik, for married couples usually do not live with any members of the family, except for a short period after they marry. This situation is common in the mestizo world, for a husband's brother visits his house and stays overnight without any trouble. It also became part of a new situation in the life of migrants to the cities for the resident family to accept their male relatives in their houses and help them to find a job. It was Daniel who invited his younger brother to his house and offered him a job as a construction worker under his own supervision. Trifena faced a new situation, which she interpreted according to a mestizo cultural code not the Tzotzil code used in Chibtik. Her other failures were a result of this misunderstanding. She had to pay a high price for it.

Last but not least, 'what is at stake' in all those conflicting explanatory models? As I mentioned before, we are inclined to give two answers to this question: one ethnographical and the other meta-ethnographical. The 'ethnography' of the social interests has already been done. What cries out for explanation is the meta-ethnography or, to follow Kleinman a meta-explanatory model. I would like to argue that, in order to work out such a model, we need what Wittgenstein called *übersichtliche Darstellung*, a figure which 'describes our form of presentation, the way we see things' (Wittgenstein 1985: 24), a perspicuous representation of the hermeneutic situation of Trifena. I think that such a representation of her odyssey of the last fours years can be found in a metaphor drawn from the poem by Blake: 'The Marriage of Heaven and Hell'. In one of the scenes of the story a narrator's soul becomes an object in a fight between black and white spiders:

> By degrees we beheld the infinite Abyss, fiery as the smoke of a burning city; beneath us at an immense distance was the sun, black but shining; round it were fiery tracks on which revolv'd vast spiders, crawling after their prey; which flew or rather swum in the infinite deep, in the most terrific shapes of animals sprung from corruption and the air was full of them, and seemed composed of them; these are Devils. And are called Powers of the air, I now asked my companion which was my eternal lot? He said, between the black and white spiders (Blake 1988: 41).

The life history of Trifena can be understood as a constant battle between different explanatory models embedded in the social experience of multiple agents, who have endeavoured to heal her soul. Protestant members of her family believe that she is either 'possessed' or is being 'punished'. More traditional family members consider her as 'chosen' by God, who sends her messages 'telling' her that she should be a *j'ilol* or a medicine-woman. The national, 'modern' doctor sees her as a victim of a neurological trauma and has tried to cure her by pharmaceutical means. Trifena's brother, more 'scientifically' and 'pragmatically' oriented, experiments with all the methods available. The anthropologist's explanatory model expresses a Western cliché, as neat as useless: 'You have to confront it, you have to ask him for a divorce...' Shall we escape a question: Who's explanatory model is a right one? Shall we escape it because we are relativists? Or perhaps ask: For whom is this question important? (Raatzsch 1993: 139)

There are two differences between Trifena's lot and Blake's vision. The 'spiders' that struggle about Trifena's fate do not understand each other and do not divide themselves into black and white. Blake could also escape his fate and jump out of the spiders' battle. Trifena's life, stigmatised by a severe illness, which has erased her personal autonomy, is doomed to it forever.

Notes

1. Chiapas is one of the three Mexican states with the highest concentration of indigenous people constituting 24.9 per cent of the state's population (see map in Figure 11.2). 16.1 per cent out of this number speak Chol, 1.4 per cent Kanjobal, 36.3 per cent Tzeltal, 48 per cent Tojolabal, 1.0 per cent Mam, 33.8 per cent Tzotzil, 4.7 per cent Zoque and 1.9 per cent some other languages like Lacandon, Kakchiquel, Mocho (Agenda Estadistica Chiapas 1996: 166). A religious mosaic presents a similar Babel's Tower: In 2000 there was only 63.82 per cent of Catholics in the state. Chenalho', Trifena's township has only 16.77 per cent of Roman Catholics. The percentage of the historical Protestants is much higher and equals to 34.92 per cent. To the Mormons, Jehovah's Witnesses and the Adventists corresponds a smaller fraction of 1.79 per cent. The rest of the inhabitants of Chenalho' (46.51 per cent) are identified as people with 'no religion', 'other religion' and 'not specified' (Rivera 2003).
2. I tried to mention some of the cures and interpretations she underwent. For the sake of the argument I omitted many visits she received, undertaken by different foreigners, (among others Aldona Jacorzynska, my sister; Magdalena Jacorzynska, my wife; María Cristina Manca, an Italian anthropologist; Steffani Behrend, a German student from Berlin; Ana Ovalle, a Spanish psychologist from Salamanca; Kenia Martins Alves, a Brasilian anthropologist). All of them had their own views on Trifena's illness and interacted with her trying to help and understand. The interpretations of those visitors together with those already mentioned in my case study constitute a rich ideological mosaic reflecting the conditions of life for a large part of Chiapanec Indians.

References

Agenda Estadistica Chiapas. 1996. *Hacienda*. Chiapas, México: Hacienda.

Ayora Díaz, I. S. 1998. 'Globalization, Rationality and Medicine: Local Medicine's Struggle for Recognition in the Highlands of Chiapas', *Urban Anthropology and Studies of Cultural Systems and World Economic Development* 27(2): 165–195.

Beltran, A.G. 1986. *Antropología médica*. México: CIESAS (Centro de Investigaciones y Estudios Superiores en Antropología Social).

Black, M. 1962. 'Metaphors', in M. Black, *Models and Metaphors. Studies in Language and Philosophy*. New York: Cornell University Press, 25–47.

Blake W. 1988. 'The Marriage of Heaven and Hell', in *The Complete Poetry & Prose of William Blake*. New York: Anchor Book, Doubleday, 33–45.

Clifford, J. 1986. 'On Ethnographic Allegory', in J. Clifford and G.E. Marcus (eds) *Writing Culture. The Poetics and Politics of Ethnography*. Berkeley: University of California Press, 99–121.

Freyermuth, G. 2000. '"Morir en Chenalho". Género, etnia y generación. Factores constijtutivos del riesgo durante la maternidad' (In process).

Good, B.J. 1994. *Medicine, Rationality, and Experience: An Anthropological Perspective*. Cambridge: Cambridge University Press.

Holland, W. 1963. *Medicina Maya en los Altos de Chiapas*. Mexico: INI (Instituto Nacional Indigenista).

Janzen, J.M. 1978. *The Quest for Therapy: Medical Pluralism in Lower Zaire*. Berkeley: University of California Press.

Kleinman, A. 1980. *Patients and Healers in the Context of Culture; An Exploration of the Borderland between Anthropology, Medicine, and Psychitary*. Berkeley: University of California Press.

——1995. *Writing at the Margin: Discourse between Anthropology and Medicine*. Berkeley: University of California Press.

Köhler, U. 1974. *Cambio social dirigido en Los Altos de Chiapas*. Mexico: INI (Instituto Nacional Indigenista).

——1995. *Choninbal Ch'ulelal- Alma Vendida. Elementos fundamentales de la cosmología y religión mesoamericanas en una oración maya-tzotzil*. Mexico: UNAM (Universidad Nacional Autónoma de México).

Lakoff, G. and M. Johnson. 1980. *Metaphors We live By*. Chicago and London: University of Chicago Press.

Laughlin, M.R. 1975. The Great Tzotzil Dictionary of San Lorenzo Zinacantán. *Smithsonian Contribuitons to Anthropology*. No. 19. Washington: Smithsonian Institute Press.

Lupton, D. 1994. *Medicine as Culture*. London: Sage.

Nichter, M. and M. Nichter. 1996. *Anthropology and International Health: Asian Case Studies*. London: Routledge.

Raatzsch, R. 1993. 'How not to Speak on Wittgenstein and Social Science', in R. Raatzsch and P. Philip (eds) *Essays on Wittgenstein. Working Papers from the Wittgenstein Archives at the University of Bergen*. No. 6. Bergen: University of Bergen, 127–153.

Ricoeur, P. 1979. 'The Metaphorical Process as Cognition. Imagination and Feeling', in S. Sacks (ed.) *On Metaphor*. Chicago: The University of Chicago Press, 141–158.

Rivera, F.C. et al. 2003. Diversidad religiosa y conflicto en Chiapas. Intereses utopias y realidades. Mexico: CIESAS, CESMECA, PROIMMSE

Schulte, J. 2001. *Wittgenstein. Eine Einführung*. Stuttgart: Philipp Reclam Jr.

Wittgenstein, L. 1985. *Bemerkungen ueber Frazers Golden Bough*. Mexico: Universidad Nacional Autónoma de México.

12

Epilogue
Multiple Medical Realities:
Reflections from Medical Anthropology

Imre Lázár and Helle Johannessen

The papers in this volume all convey plurality in medicine. The perspectives differ from one study to another and plurality is exposed and explored at different levels and in different contexts. And yet some patterns seem to cut across all the differences. From the health-seeking behaviour of Tamil refugees in the north of Norway to treatment of mental illness in Ghana and Mexico, and from psychologists in Hungary to homoeopaths in London, a very broad concept of health and healing seems to be of importance. All papers show that sick persons, families and healers interpret symptoms as signs of social and spiritual disturbance. In fact, social and spiritual aspects of sickness and healing seem to be generally acknowledged and acted upon, a feature which questions the hegemonic concept of sickness as a physical problem primarily calling for physical interventions. A pattern connecting people in all the localities studied is that whatever sickness they suffer, the problem is not only understood as a problem of the physical body, but also as one of the self. And strategies to get well likewise concern not only well-being of the body, but also restoration of the self and of relations with others, be they neighbours, spirits, saints, or God.

Plural use of medicine and choices between different forms of medicine among practitioners and patients seem to be informed by whatever concepts of health and healing are employed by the person taking action. Some practitioners employ technologies of healing from different traditions in order to cover a wide range of issues considered relevant to healing. Others believe that they have found a technology that encompasses multiple aspects of sickness and healing, and prefer that to more monistic technologies. Yet others practise a rather narrow form of treatment leaving other aspects of sickness to be treated by other kinds of healer. The sick persons and their families do, however, all seem to seek relief for the corporeal body as well as for the social and spiritual body by attending a broad range of healthcare options or holistic technologies.

One may wonder to what extent these findings have validity beyond the relatively few persons represented in the papers of this volume. Have the anthropologists in their search for medical pluralism and diversity focused on small exotic minorities of persons who go doctor-shopping for holism or who provide personally constructed eclectic health technologies? Or do the patterns connecting these studies also connect to a wider range of humankind? As shown in Buda et al.'s quantitative study, plural use of medicine is indeed not restricted to exotic minorities; rather, plural use seems to be a general feature in Europe and the United States (Buda et al, this volume), and from other studies we know it is also widespread in South America, Africa and Asia (Koss-Chioino et al. 2003, Nichter and Lock 2002, Whyte et al. 2003). These studies from other parts of the world likewise demonstrate a multifaceted conception of sickness and healing among local people in the search for, or provision of, healthcare. We thus seem to face a general, perhaps universal, understanding of sickness as much more than the physical pathology dominating disease models of biomedicine, science and official public discourse.

The universal presence of concepts and praxis of holistic health deserves proper attention and compels us to ask a number of questions. Some relate to the ontology of body and self, and thus of the objects and subjects of medicine, as well as to anthropology. Other issues concern relations of structure and power between state-supported medicine and politically marginalised medicines.

Multiple realities of body and self

In the introductory chapter of this volume, Johannessen urges a concept of the complex body that incorporates the eyes that 'see' and the discourse in which the body is articulated, as well as individual and political body praxis. She also points to the evidence regarding selves as flexible actors in a constant struggle for social recognition, as well as evidence of the complex body in need of care as a significant factor in that struggle.

The concepts of complex bodies and flexible selves could lead to anticipations that the plurality of body and self reflects a plethora of discursive forms, and are thus primarily constructions that do not necessarily refer to 'real' bodies and selves. But we would like to turn these anticipations upside down and suggest that the evidence of medical plurality be taken seriously, since we consider the discursive plethora to be a reflection of complexity in the body per se. Anthropology has for too long relied on duplex epistemologies that allowed members of the profession to praise cultural diversity and relativity in epistemologies, but at the same time to rest secure in Western scientific epistemology as the 'true' conceptions of reality (cf. Pels 1999). If we take seriously the idea that the dominant scientific epistemology is also culturally formed and anchored in a certain 'perspective' that leaves out more than it encompasses, this epistemology is not a priori superior to other local epistemologies. This means that it is not necessarily a more 'true' representation of reality than other epistemologies. The worldwide presence of epistemologies and praxis forms regarding body and self, sickness and healing, as multidimensional phenomena including the social, spiritual and biological calls for a consideration of the ontology of the body.

As Lock and Scheper-Hughes (1990) has pointed out, medical anthropology can potentially be a much more radical undertaking than just the study of 'other' medical systems and practices. It may be a messenger of knowledge of the body, health and illness as culturally constructed, negotiated and renegotiated in a dynamic process through time and space. This way medical anthropology may play the role of transcultural mediator in a dialogue between different medical realities.

Or versus *and*: exclusive ontologies or multiple social realities

Ontology in its Platonistic sense is a description of *essential reality*, as opposed to what one can see or what one can know. This hidden claim to universal truth is part of the exclusive hegemonism of modernism. The legitimation of biomedicine's monopolistic drive stems from the ontological axiom that Nature/Truth is Universal and independent of Time and Space. According to Gordon's depiction of the basic assumptions of bioreductionist naturalism, the human body as biomedical object becomes *Nature* as distinct from the 'Supernatural', mere Matter as opposed to Spirit. This bodily Nature is independent of human consciousness. As Nature, it is separate from culture and morality. The analytic approach creates *Atomism*, where the Part is independent of and primordial to the Whole (Gordon 1988). In naturalistic ontology the human body as natural medical object is disengaged from society, culture, emotion, and particular time and place.

The naturalistic ontology may even gain support from cultural anthropology, including ecological, ethological, sociobiological, developmental, Marxist, and cultural materialist objectivism. When theory and practice are embodied in the framework of materialistic and statistical objectivity, one may easily oppose the classical 'Benedictine' notion that 'abnormality' and 'normality' are culturally defined categories. This is reflected by the proposed analytic framework that combines the emic perspective of ethnomedicine with the etic measures of bioscience as stated by Browner et al. (1988). This medical anthropological approach finds a stable base in the biosciences for anchoring the diversity in the reference of normal values and standards of nature. The addressing of diverse cultural realities with psychobiological standards behind them hopes to generate valuable new interpretations for cross-cultural, comparative studies of human physiological processes, exploring how such processes are perceived, and what culture-specific behaviours are produced by these perceptions (Browner et al. 1988). This particular anthropological attitude is more common in medical schools where medical anthropology is taught as part of the behavioural sciences.

The rigid naturalist framework may be loosened, overcoming the Cartesian dualism by way of the mind/body concept. Social psychophysiology may dissolve the borders between natural, social and cultural phenomena connecting mind and body, but this is a sort of extension of bodily 'neurophysiological' Nature in the direction of cultural, social and psychic phenomena instead of a spiritualisation of human suffering and healing. The social-psychophysiological mechanisms may play the role of a hermeneutic in the case of symbolic healing and the pathophysiology of culture-bound diseases (Lázár 1987). Psychophysiologist explanatory models are abundant regarding voodoo deaths, as well as painful healing ceremonies and initiation rites (Frecska and Kulcsár 1989). Psychoneuroimmunology is one of the emerging social-psychophysiological explanatory models uncovering the 'secrets' of exotic healing ceremonies and culture-bound syndromes (Lázár 1994).

Placebo as common key to different medical realities

The placebo/nocebo theory may offer keys to the black box of unconventional medicine without disturbing the naturalist ontology. Nevertheless, Peters is right to point out that dismissing human factors with a powerful influence on health and treatments as mere placebo responses or the result of pious fraud is no longer satisfactory (Peters 2001). The question of placebo raises the question of social reality instead of ontology since placebo and nocebo are culture bound and context dependent. The placebo's main content is often anticipated to be 'belief'. This extended anthropological notion of placebo includes 'pill, potion and procedure', and their context, and thus points to why multiple social realities instead of universal and exclusive ontologies help us to accept the diversity of healing. Nevertheless, for the sake of ontological reassurance we shall search out a definitive explanatory mechanism in the hope that psycho-neurophysiological patterns will throw light on the highly context-dependent influences of healers. In order to explore the deep layers of placebo and nocebo effect, we require knowledge of physical, cultural, social and economic context (Helman 2001). But a (social-)psychophysiological approach helps to reintegrate the most subtle social and cultural influences into the naturalist framework. Mind represents these influences in patterns of neurocircuit activity and the neuropeptide language of the unconscious. When we create a sharp distinction between the reductionist scientific approach to illness causation (in which simple processes give rise to more complex ones: so-called upward causation) and the holistic approach (with its downward causation model), we may remain within the naturalistic paradigm. Downward causation is when higher-order systems control lower-order systems within the body. The control is thought to go from mind, which includes social and cultural meaning, through the central nervous system to bodily function (Sperry 1987). As complex systems are selforganising, very small changes in the dynamics of the system can lead to the emergence of quite new organising principles, where thoughts, feelings and beliefs are organising principles that lead to the emergence of control functions within the body as a whole. Control, hope, laughter and a feeling of success are markers of effective and active coping, enhancing psychoimmunological competence, while learned helplessness, giving up, resignation, defeat, loss of control and depression may depress immunity. But all these events are played out in a naturalistic scene. Since unconventional medicine may enhance hope, optimism and a feeling of control, it may strengthen aspecific psychophysiological protective processes. In this way the psychobiological holism of mind and body integrates social, psycho- and physiological discursive levels in one neurophysiological framework wired by neuroendocrine-immune informational pathways. It is a sort of extension of the bodily cosmos to the social world, exploring how the person embodies cultural and social influences.

This is why Samuel's model offers an important additional step towards a more open ontology protecting the position of rationalism. In his ecological approach, any explanation has to be phrased in terms of mind, body and social and physical environment *as a whole*. The wide range of context-dependent *states* of the mind-body-society-environment complex or *modal states* is no longer a simple extension of psychophysiological machinery, but must be evaluated as *cultural* states and 'as a repertoire of *personal* states possessed by each individual, and learned and internalised during their lifetime' (Samuel, this volume).

Downward from beyond

In the ontological framework of metaphysics, a spiritual framework is not a form of bio-psycho-social medicine; it is a radically extended version of the Engelian paradigm. In the bio-psycho-social-spiritual model, the biological, the psychological, the social and the spiritual are merely distinct dimensions of the person, and no one aspect can be disaggregated from the whole.

In a modernist 'antinomic' framework, the opposite choice is – as Ulbæk (1994) writes – the *alternativist ontology of unconventional medicine*, which may be classified as one based on metaphysical commitments where the paranormal reality of bioenergetic therapy, retroactive and intercessory prayer, homoeopathy, chakra therapy, neoshamanism and faith healing are put out of the sphere of physical reality by means of two readings: either physical reality is included within paranormal reality, in which case it is a subset of paranormal reality, or paranormal reality is an outer sphere surrounding physical reality without any claims on behalf of physical reality. The practice of Táltos healers and the case of the distance healing of a tumour patient by her son offer challenging examples of this alternativist ontology in Lázár's paper in the present volume.

According to Benor (1990), *spiritual healing* is thought to include approaches that involve the intentional influence of one or more persons upon another living system without utilising known physical means of intervention. Distance healing also includes approaches commonly referred to as 'prayer'. Its importance cannot be overestimated, since in the United Kingdom there are more distance healers than there are therapists in any other branch of complementary and alternative medicine (Astin et al. 2000).

Spiritual means of therapy and metaphysical ontology are not denied at all in the world of healing. A national survey conducted in the United States in 1996 found that 82 per cent of Americans believed in the healing power of prayer and 64 per cent felt that physicians should pray with patients who request it (Wallis 1996). Religious commitment, attending worship, prayer, seeking and asking forgiveness from those important to one, and reading Holy Writ may play a role in illness prevention, in coping with illness and in recovery (Matthews et al. 1998). As Astin's (1998) research has shown, the majority of those using alternative medicine are well educated, report poor health status, and use alternative medicine not so much as a result of dissatisfaction with conventional medicine but largely because they find alternative healthcare to be more congruent with their own values, beliefs, and philosophical orientations toward health and life.

If conscious intent in the form of prayer can act retroactively on distant persons and affect past events, this may challenge the naturalist ontology in its very foundations. Leibovici provoked and tested the vigilance and sensitivity of the scientific community with the question of whether one can believe a study that seems methodologically correct but tests something that is completely outside people's conception (or model) of the physical world. He published an intriguing study questioning conventional notions of time, space, prayer, consciousness and causality. The randomised, controlled, double-blind, parallel-group study (prayer versus no prayer) included 3393 septic patients and considered the hypothesis that 'retroactive' prayer, offered between four and ten years later affects outcomes. Of the pre-selected outcomes, mortality was similar in both groups, yet length of stay in hospital and duration of fever were shorter with prayer (Leibovici 2001). Controlled clinical trials, reviews and meta-analyses of distance healing and prayer also reported positive findings (Astin et al. 2000). Other opinions seem to be more critical with regard to the statistical validity (Courcey 2001, Kaptchuk 2001).

Games without frontiers

When ontologies – be they canonised metaphysical or rational naturalist – have a strong claim to hegemony and dominance, medical pluralism becomes a war zone. The persecution of traditional healers on religious or biomedical legal grounds may be a sign of this hegemonism. In Western societies biomedicine has occupied a niche in modern life in which its hegemony regarding healing seems to be taken for granted. This hegemony is based on its increasingly high-tech assisted and evidence-based *efficacy*, on the dominant 'naturalist' and 'positivist' assumptions that bring to biomedicine the air of success associated with the natural sciences (Gordon 1988), and on the spirit of the Enlightenment that frames the historical development of scientific medicine.

During the historical period of modernity, formerly conventional healing traditions have become unconventional means of healing and are by now considered marginal. The umbrella definition of unconventional therapies reflects the powergame content of this medical pluralism as 'alternative medicine is a broad domain of healing resources that encompass all health systems, modalities and practices and their accompanying theories and beliefs, other than those intrinsic to the politically dominant health system of a particular society or culture in a given historical period' (Monckton et al. 1999: 15). The same issue of the power content of hegemony is reflected in another definition of alternative medicine, where alternative medicine is any sort of health/disease-related intervention, method or system that challenges the commonly accepted medical status quo or the bureaucratic priorities of the dominant professional healthcare in a given age and in a given society (Dossey and Swyers 1994). These phrases reflect the fact that alternative medicine, with its different ontological content, represents a challenging counter-culture and covers ritual antistructure, just as it did in the past, too.

The historical waves of modernisation seem to repeat their attacks on obscured, sometimes magical, healing traditions. In sixteenth century Hungary, the Protestant modernisation was reflected by criminalisation of magical healing, while the Habsburg Empire's oppressive Catholic acculturation increased the pressure of accusations against folk healers, who were regarded as fraudulent and ineffective practitioners (Klaniczay 1990). Although the ideology of the class struggle slowly disappeared during the decades of 'socialism in being', there was a period when these spiritual or traditional healers were seen as representing a danger to the 'enlightened, scientific' dialectical materialist worldview and political system. Consequently, they were victims of political persecution in Hungary during the 1950s and early 1960s (Gryneus 2002).

In the nineteenth century there were various waves of medical counter-culture rebels in the United States. These involved organised opposition from Thomsonians, Grahamites, homoeopaths, hydropaths, mesmerists, osteopaths, chiropractors and Christian Scientists (Kaptchuk and Eisenberg

2001). The fight included rhetoric, legislative moves and the use of cultural symbols, with the counter-healers showing genius in protesting against the dominant order concerning its therapeutics as well as its political and religious ideas (Starr 1983). This traditional opposition between modernist and alternativist healers remained unchanged during the modernist twentieth. century. Mainstream journals of biomedicine, such as the *New England Journal of Medicine*, warned physicians to protect their patients against 'fraudulent exploitation' by alternative medicine. Even in the mid-1980s one could read a dispatch from the battlefield in which 'one government report estimated that in 1970 quackery cost $1–2 billion a year and today, in 1984, the cost probably totals at least $10 billion' (US Government 1984). Representatives of the power centres of the evidence-based machinery of medical knowledge have a different view of a conciliatory common framework for statistically verifiable truth. They state: 'There is no alternative medicine. There is only scientifically proven, evidence-based medicine supported by solid data or unproven medicine, for which scientific evidence is lacking. Whether a therapeutic practice is "Eastern" or "Western", is unconventional or mainstream, or involves mind-body techniques or molecular genetics is largely irrelevant except for historical purposes and cultural interest' (Fontanarosa and Lundberg 1998).

As modernism turned into postmodernism, the medical hegemony situation changed radically. The recent widespread and growing interest in alternative medicine also represents a dramatic reconfiguration of medical pluralism.

Ecology of symbolic worlds

How can we free ourselves from the *dia*-bolic binary trap of naturalism/ metaphysicism without denying the ontology of Nature and/or Supernature? An ecological framework offers a bypass route to avoid a decision.

The landscape of medical *memes* may uncover the ecodynamic relationships between social realities of healing. The ecodynamism of different patterns of medical memes may result in dominant versus submissive interrelationships, neutral ways of coexistence or symbiotic mutualism. The narrative of Trifena, the Maya lady in Jarcorzynski's paper, proves that the plethora of different competing healing methods, such as biomedical anti-parasitic pharmacological therapy, psychopharmacons, prayer, traditional Maya rituals, herbs, exorcism and Pentecostal spiritism, may intrude into one patient's history.

The ecorelationship between traditional, spiritual, biomedical and other memes of healing is described by Krause in her paper, where herbalists, bonesetters, traditional midwives, Muslim healers such as mallams and marabouts, possession priests such as the *akomfo* among the Akan, Tigare and Mami Wata shrines, and a variety of Christian healers and prophets work in a very diverse medical landscape. Their different methods create a social and cultural ranking of medical practices as a result of competition and supportive networking. But we find the same challenging diversity of medical realities in the United Kingdom, Hungary and Mexico. The postmodern landscape of healing shows a negotiable, multiple, local, modest and provisional medical reality.

The above findings support the idea that people do not necessarily think in terms of mutually exclusive alternatives (as implied by the term 'alternative medicine'). Although consumers in the 'health plaza' are strongly influenced by the health media and the state-supported or professional ideological hierarchy, they nevertheless have their own personal affinities based on their own value and belief systems to prioritise and to prefer one form of treatment to another. They do not try out therapies at random, although the particular configurations of the hierarchies of services consumed vary from one person to another, and perhaps from one time to another for an individual.

Aspecific health protective factors, psychoimmunological mechanisms and expectation-attribution or placebo effect are legitimating explanations for a scientific approach regarding the not-yet-understood aspects of unconventional medicine, but they cover up rather than provide insight into the working mechanism. Different needs and expectations sustain different patterns of memes. The same consumer of given medical memes may turn to different healers without any internal conflict, cognitive dissonance or loss of scientific commitment. This ecosystem of healing practices is itself a plural medical system embedded in the wider social, technological and natural, or even supernatural, reality.

Some of the consumers of these diverse healing practices exhibiting special cosmology and ontology do not think much about the 'hermetic' world behind the medicament offered, and as Barry shows (this volume), their preconceptions are those of *normative biomedical patients* with dualistic and mechanistic views of their bodies. Use of different healing services does not, therefore, necessarily mean plural philosophy and multiple medical reality. But we cannot speak of multiple medical reality even in the case of *committed homoeopathic patients* possessing a different view of their bodies, health and healing through their embodied experiences with homoeopathy and their interactions with homoeopaths. They may elect homoeopathy exclusively.

But there are many who seek help utilising a conscious, complementing approach and postmodern pragmatic eclecticism. They seldom give information to their biomedical doctor about their alternative choices, and this may be interpreted as the avoidance of conflict between the different competing fields.

In the network of multiple medical realities

Although the Schutzian concept of multiple reality is not itself postmodern and does not challenge the unitary (naturalist or metaphysical) ontological frame, the postmodern approach is unviable without this Schutzian term. According to Schutz (1973) it is the meaning of our experiences and not the ontological structure of the objects which constitutes reality. The diversity of medical cosmologies may be interpreted using Schutz's social phenomenological approach of various finite provinces of meanings. His thesis about relevance may be extended to medical metaphors, representations and knowledge as well; that relevance is not inherent in nature as such is the result of the selective and interpretive activity of man within nature or observing nature. When patients enter any of these provinces of different medical meanings, such as the clinical realities of Traditional Chinese Medicine, homoeopathy or Ayurvedic medicine, this may be seen as a radical choice between different worlds. Each field may contain distinctive logical, temporal, corporal and social dimensions. Nevertheless, these terrains are permeable, and patients adopt the attitudes of scientist or religious believer *within* the world of working. Schutz (1973) helps us to understand how patients may 'surf' through different, more-or-less incompatible medical worlds without any cognitive dissonance, because when a patient believes that something is true and real, he/she automatically gives it the status of reality. In these diverse medical 'lifeworlds' experiences become social along the constraints and rules of symbolic healing (Dow 1986). These experiential 'worlds' are not external or objective worlds, but rather are attitudes toward the world exhibiting different degrees of attention to external reality, different forms of spontaneity, different experiences of the self, time, sociality and so on (Schutz 1973).

During this journey among different symbolic worlds one may go beyond the limits of the world within one's actual reach and transgress the paramount reality of everyday life. We must bear in mind that subjective social reality is always an interpretation of the 'real' world. Medical ontologies appear for patients and healers as narrative representations of facts and situations explaining reality, and give every element a logical place of its own in the lifeworld. In this jungle of metaphors, explanatory models and medical representations, one can change from one medical reality to another, different, sometimes incompatible, one. As Johannessen (this volume) emphasises, the various medical realities and cosmologies do not exist as the coexistence of separate and independent sociocultural systems of medicine, but are embedded in networks based on affinal organising principles linking the medical narratives and forms of praxis to issues of power and social relations. The dissolving of a single modernist medical narrative has formed an increased awareness of medical pluralism. The concept of multiple medical reality may be conceived of as a postmodern phenomenon, since postmodernism emphasises multiplicity, plurality, fragmentation and indeterminacy, which are embodied in this networking. The network approach may dissolve the dyadic frontiers as 'the old cultural war of a dominant culture versus heretical rebellion in politics and religion as well as medicine has begun to transform into a recognition of postmodern multiple narratives' (Kaptchuk 2001).

Why does the tolerant 'anti-*anti*' postmodern attitude nevertheless generate *anti*structure to modernity? Postmodern scholars aim at documenting representations of multiple realities of laypersons as real and existentially true ways of knowing. As Johannessen (this volume) writes, this approach as part of the postmodern rebellion against science implied revolt against the hegemonic status of scientific knowledge, i.e., knowledge that was based on a detached, disembodied objectification of diseases, patients, nature, and much more. In much postmodern medical anthropology, the plethora of experiences was acknowledged and discussed as part of existence and as part of the lifeworld of individuals, but not as part of larger social and cultural structures.

The category of the modern is closely linked to the concept of universality. The universality of disease categories frees the disease entities from local social, cultural and individual psychological contexts, while the local philosophies of healing recontextualise the disease in the framework of unconventional medicine.

Medicine and healing

What lessons can be learned by professionals in the researching and practice of medicine from discussions of body and self in medical pluralism? Although the multiple medical realities embodied in the heterogeneity of healing and the plurality of discourses, in institutions and forms of praxis available to the individual, may induce anxiety and sometimes frustration and anger in biomedical experts, a number of important aspects stand out as important and constructive for the development of medicine in the twenty-first century.

First of all, Buda et al.'s paper (this volume) as well as other research proves that we have to give up the former belief that alternative, complementary and traditional forms of medicine are primarily used by credulous people who, out of ignorance, tend to avoid modern, scientifically based forms of medicine. Just the opposite is true. Alternative forms of healing seem to be mostly used by those who visit medical doctors more frequently; people with chronic or severe forms of disease thus tend to use a wide range of the available possibilities of healing illnesses and maintaining good health. If state-authorised medical professionals and the scientific community want to sustain the dominant position occupied at present and keep their role in gatekeeping and advising patients about their needs, it is necessary for them to become familiarised with complementary and alternative forms of medicine. Those in favour of keeping the status quo power structures anxiously warn that if biomedical experts do not know alternative medicine, it is likely that the provision of complementary and alternative medicine will occur through a growing network of parallel healthcare providers involving larger numbers of non-medically qualified practitioners. One important way of promoting familiarisation with unconventional forms of medicine is through the integration of complementary and alternative medicine into the medical curriculum; this would promote contact with, and networks including, those outside the circle of conventional medicine and the medical schools. Such contact could be an important step in the integration of complementary and alternative medicine with other medical services.

This process may lessen the anxiety of medical doctors, but cannot reduce the multiplicity of proliferating medical realities, because this multiplicity is fed and supported by patients, families and healers that seek alternative forms of therapy in concordance with a multiplicity and heterogeneity of realities. The dynamism of this eternal repopulation of non-official niches in the world of healing partly has its roots in the antistructure of permanent cognitive rebellion against determinative rationality. It may be necessary for medical students to learn how to deal with unconventional medicine as a different reality instead of learning a reduced range of domesticated unconventional therapies censored by way of evidence-based methodology.

Medical anthropology has an important task in helping to integrate knowledge gained from different elective courses of unconventional medicine. Knowledge of the close relations between culture and healing is essential in critical clinical thinking and may help to control medical behaviours and ideologies being taken for granted. This may be achieved by a syncretic synthesis of modern and postmodern, bioscience and social anthropology. The teaching of medical anthropology in the medical curriculum – it has been compulsory in several medical schools throughout Europe since the mid-1990s – imposes responsibility for making a compromise between a modern science and its postmodern narrative offered by medical anthropology. The preclinical period of the medical curriculum, when assertiveness, commitment and professional group identity are built up with high mental loading and stress at a liminal stage of a *rite de passage*, may be the right time for medical anthropology to be incorporated into the education of health professionals. Since the biomedical gaze and the dominant research trend (including the new game of evidence-based medicine) can – despite all its expertise and accuracy – cover only part of the heterogeneous relations of body, self and environment, teaching medical anthropology and unconventional medicine may extend the horizon of interest and multiply medical identity.

Since any form of local medicine offers only one perspective (one discourse in the Foucauldian sense) that articulates only a small part of the heterogeneous plethora of reality, the 'multilingual' hermeneutic turn of medical anthropological interest in unconventional medicine may help to expand the range of available and known discourses. In a plural medical system the skills of critical and self-reflective judgment are most important.

We must bear in mind that one person may shift through radically different realities or cosmologies of his body that are embodied in variable metaphors and explanatory models of his suffering, as in the case of Jacorcynski's Maya patient or a biomedically trained homoeopathic healer using acupuncture, therapeutic touch or prayer in his healing arsenal. The chaos of contradictory explanatory models may disturb the sick person's creation of meaning in the midst of his suffering, and he may find himself lost without cooperating helpers. This is why collaboration is urged in the training of medical doctors regarding alternative medicine. This calls for a different acknowledgement of medical pluralism on a personal level and on the local scale. We need a theoretical framework for understanding patterns in the multiple and contradictory experiences and practices of body and self in which one individual engages, and which is found in local society everywhere. Medical anthropology may offer tools to handle this challenge without disturbing the processes of identity formation, in which evaluation, selection and personal and cultural self-perceptions may be integrated. The culturally sensitive approach may offer an educative and safe process of medical self-exploration diminishing the risks of crisis along the way. In that sense it is similar to stress inoculation processes as a sort of controlled crisis. Medical anthropology may build antistructure into the developing structure, making medical identity stronger, just as stress-inoculation makes personality stronger and immunised against stressors.

Being familiar with multiple medical realities gives doctors and the health profession an opportunity to bring together the strengths, and to counterbalance the weaknesses, inherent in different systems of healthcare. This means to enhance the skills of orientation and openness in fields of different medical worlds, as proposed by Jonas when he urges that medical and nursing education concerning complementary and alternative practice should include information about the philosophical paradigm, scientific foundation, training provision, practice, and evidence of safety and efficacy of the discipline or disciplines in question (Jonas 1998). Future medicine should not only rely on research into genes and molecular biology (smaller and smaller entities of the body), but should also include an approach in the opposite direction, one where the body is conceived of as an entity deeply related to, and dependent on, social, cultural and psychological fields of relations.

Finally, two laws of healing must remain unaltered in the changing cosmos of diverse medical subuniversa. These are 'Nil nocere' and 'Salus aegroti suprema lex esto', 'Do no harm' because 'The patient's interests must always come first'.

References

Astin, J.A. 1998. 'Why Patients Use Alternative Medicine. Results of a National Study', *Journal of the American Medical Association* 279: 1548–1553.

Astin, J.A., E. Harkness and D. Ernst. 2000. 'The Efficacy of "Distant Healing": A Systematic Review of Randomized Trials', *Annals of Internal Medicine* 132(11): 903–910.

Benor, D. 1990. 'Survey of spiritual healing research', *Complementary Medical Research* 1990(4): 9–33.

Browner, C.H., B.R. Ortiz de Montellano and A.J. Rubel. 1988. 'A Methodology for Cross-cultural Ethnomedical Research', *Current Anthropology* 29(5): 681–702.

Courcey, K. 2001. 'Distant Healing', *Annals of Internal Medicine* 134(6): 532–32.

Dossey, L. and J.P. Swyers. 1994. *Introduction to Alternative Medicine: Expanding Medical Horizons*. Washington, DC: US Government Printing Office, NIH, 94–166.

Dow, J. 1986. 'Universal Aspects of Symbolic Healing', *American Anthropologist* 88: 56–69.

Fontanarosa, P.B. and G.D. Lundberg. 1998. 'Alternative Medicine meets Science', Editorial, *Journal of the American Medical Association* 280: 1618–1619.

Frecska E. and Z. Kulcsár. 1989. 'Social Bonding in the Modulation of the Physiology of Ritual Trance', *Ethos* 17(1): 70–87.

Gordon, D.R. 1988. 'Tenacious Assumptions in Western Medicine', in M. Lock and D. Gordon (eds) *Biomedicine Examined*. Dordrecht: Kluwer Academic Publishers, 19–56.

Grynaeus, T. 2002. 'A fehértói javas ember tudománya' [Knowledge of the 'javas' healer from Fehértó], *Csongrádi megyei könyvtári füzetek* 23: 5–160.

Helman, C.G. 2001. 'Placebos and nocebos: the cultural construction of belief', in D. Peters (ed.) *Understanding the Placebo Effect in Complementary Medicine*. Edinburgh: Churchill, Livingstone, 3–37.

Jonas, W. 1998. 'Alternative Medicine and the Conventional Practitioner', *Journal of the American Medical Association* 279: 708–709.

Kaptchuk, T.J. 2001. 'Distant Healing', *Annals of Internal Medicine* 134(6): 532.

Kaptchuk, T.J. and D.M. Eisenberg. 2001. 'Varieties of Healing. 1: Medical Pluralism in the United States', *Annals of Internal Medicine* 135(3): 189–195.

Klaniczay, G. 1990. *The Uses of Supernatural Power*. London: Polity Press.

Koss-Chioino, J., T. Leatherman and C. Greenway (eds) 2003. *Medical Pluralism in the Andes*. London and New York.

Lázár, I. 1987. 'Role of Social-psychophysiology in Medical Antropology', paper to IBRO Social-psychophysiology Satellite Symposium, Gálosfa, Hungary, August 1987.

Lázár, I. 1994. 'Szociál-pszichoimmunológia' [Social-psychoimmunology: PNI explanatory models in medical anthropology], unpublished Ph.D. thesis, Hungarian Academy of Science.

Leibovici, L. 2001. 'Effects of Remote, Retroactive Intercessory Prayer on Outcomes in Patients with Bloodstream Infection: Randomised Controlled Trial', *British Medical Journal* 323: 1450–1451.

Lock, M. and N. Scheper-Hughes. 1990. 'A Critical-interpretive Approach in Medical Anthropology: Rituals and Routines of Discipline and Dissent', in T.M. Johnson and C.F. Sargent (eds) *Medical Anthropology. Contemporary Theory and Method.* New York: Praeger, 47–72.

Matthews, D.A., M.E. McCullough, D.B. Larson, H.G. Koenig, J.P. Swyers and M. Greenwold Milano. 1998. 'Religious Commitment and Health Status. A Review of the Research and Implications for Family Medicine', *Archives of Family Medicine* 7: 118–124.

Monckton, J., B. Belicza, W. Betz, H. Engelbart and M. van Wassenhoven (eds) 1998. *COST Action B4 – Unconventional Medicine. Final Report of the*

Management Committee 1993–98. Luxembourgh: Office for Official Publications of the European Communities.

US Government, 1984. *Quackery: A $10 Billion Scandal. A Report by the Chairman of the Subcommittee on Health and Long-term Care of the Select Committee on Aging*. House of Representatives. 98th Congress. Comm. Pub. No. 98–435. Washington, DC: U.S. Government Printing Office.

Nichter, M. and M. Lock. (eds.) 2002. *New Horizons in Medical Anthropology. Essays in Honour of Charles Leslie*. London and New York: Routledge.

Pels, P. 1999. 'Professions of Duplexity – A Prehistory of Ethical Codes in Anthropology', *Current Anthropology* 40(2): 101–136.

Peters, D. 2001. 'Preface', in D. Peters (ed.) *Understanding the Placebo Effect in Complementary Medicine*. Edinburgh: Churchill, Livingstone, i–xiv.

Schutz, A. 1973 [1945]. *Collected Papers I: The Problem of Social Reality*. Edited and introduced by M. Natanson. The Hague: Nijhoff.

Sperry, R.W. 1987. 'Structure and Significance of the Consciousness Revolution', *Journal of Mind and Behavior* 8: 37–65.

Starr, P. 1983. *The Social Transformation of American Medicine*. New York: Basic Books.

Ulbæk, I. 1994. 'Ontological Problems in Constructing Alternative Realities', in H. Johannessen, L. Launsø, S.G. Olesen and F. Staugaard (eds) *Studies in Alternative Therapy 1. Contributions from the Nordic countries*. Odense: Odense University Press and INRAT, 213–226.

Wallis, C. 1996. 'Faith and Healing: Can Prayer, Faith and Spirituality Really Improve Your Physical Health? A Growing and Surprising Body of Scientific Evidence Says They Can', *Time* 147: 58.

Whyte, S.R., S. van der Geest and A. Hardon (eds) 2003. *Social Lives of Medicines*. Cambridge Studies in Medical Anthropology. Cambridge: Cambridge University Press.

Index